Mediterranean Diet for Beginners 2024

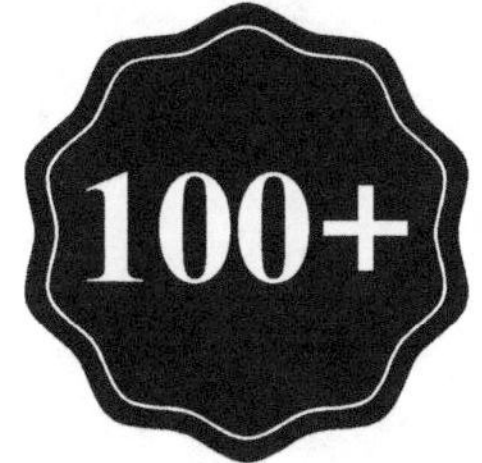

hand-picked recipes, Easy and Stress-free, made to help you build healthy eating habits.

14-day meal plan to get you started

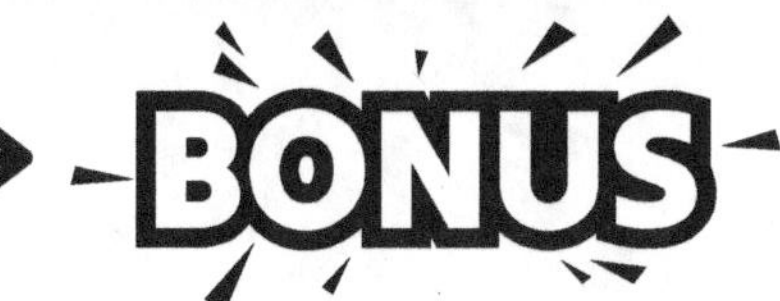

By Janie Stafford

Copyright

Disclaimer

The information provided in this book is for general informational purposes only and should not be taken as a substitute for professional medical advice.

The author and publisher make no representations or warranties about the accuracy, completeness, reliability, suitability, or availability of the content. Any reliance you place on such information is at your own risk.

The recipes, dietary advice, and lifestyle suggestions in this book are not a substitute for professional medical advice, diagnosis, or treatment. Always consult with your physician or another qualified health provider with any questions you may have regarding a medical condition.

The author and publisher disclaim any liability or loss in connection with the content provided in this book. The inclusion of product names, brands, or specific dietary recommendations does not imply endorsement or sponsorship by the author or the publisher.

Results may vary, and any diet or lifestyle change should be undertaken with careful consideration of personal health conditions and in consultation with healthcare professionals.

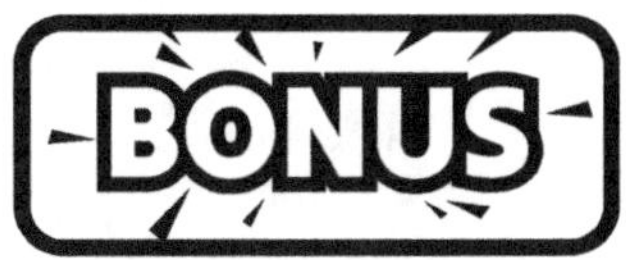 14-Day Meal Plan to get you started with MEDITERRANEAN DIET. All recipes and process for preparing are discussed later in the Book.

DAY 1

Breakfast: Crustless Quiche with Spinach and Mushrooms
Lunch: Tuna Patties Fried in Olive Oil (France)
Dinner: Garlicky Spinach and Chickpea Soup with Lemon and Pecorino Romano

DAY 2

Breakfast: Spanakopita Egg Muffins (Easy Egg Bite Recipe!)
Lunch: Bean Burgers with Garlic and Sage
Dinner: Spicy Sweet Potato Tacos

DAY 3

Breakfast: Pita Breakfast Pizza with Za'atar
Lunch: Avocado Toast with Caramelized Balsamic Onions
Dinner: Chickpea Caesar Salad with a Cheater's Dressing

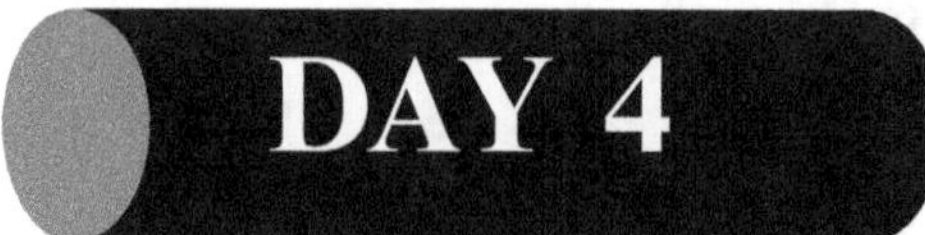

Breakfast: Healthy Blueberry Muffins (Whole Wheat!)

Lunch: Pasta Alla Puttanesca with Canned Tuna

Dinner: Marinated White Bean and Tomato Salad

DAY 5

Breakfast: Egg White Frittata with Smoked Salmon

Lunch: Avocado Salad with Cucumber and Radish

Dinner: Crispy Chickpeas and Scallops with Garlic-Harissa Oil

DAY 6

Breakfast: Asparagus Quiche

Lunch: Lebanese Hummus

Dinner: Mediterranean Quinoa Bowls with Roasted Red Pepper Sauce

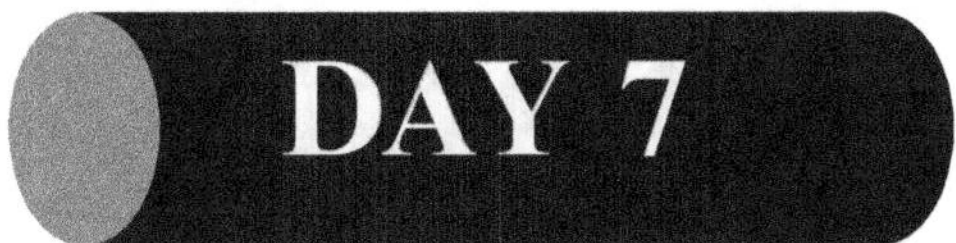

DAY 7

Breakfast: Soft Scrambled Eggs

Lunch: Garlic Soup with Egg and Croutons

Dinner: Baked Chicken and Ricotta Meatballs

DAY 8

Breakfast: Sweet Potato Hash Recipe with Za'atar and Chickpeas

Lunch: Muhammara (Roasted Red Pepper and Walnut Dip)

Dinner: Winter One-Pan Chicken and Veggies

DAY 9

Breakfast: Easy Oven Baked Eggs

Lunch: Beet and Carrot Salad with Walnuts and Goat Cheese

Dinner: Lemon Salmon with Garlic and Thyme

DAY 10

Breakfast: Breakfast Strata (Baked Egg Casserole)
Lunch: Grilled Cheese with Feta and Sun-Dried Tomatoes
Dinner: Chickpea Vegetable Coconut Curry

DAY 11

Breakfast: Leftover Mashed Potato Pancakes
Lunch: Moroccan Harira (Lentil and Chickpea Soup)
Dinner: Kale Salad with Crispy Chickpeas

DAY 12

Breakfast: Challah French Toast with Orange Honey Syrup
Lunch: Avocado Toast with Smoked Salmon, Fresh Dill, and Capers
Dinner: Sweet Potato Noodles with Almond Sauce

DAY 13

Breakfast: Egg Toast with Vegetables (Healthy Breakfast Recipe)
Lunch: Pasta Genovese in Pasta or Potato Salad or on Bread
Dinner: Blistered Green Beans with Tomatoes

DAY 14

Breakfast: Eggs Fra Diavolo
Lunch: Authentic Greek Salad
Dinner: Baked Sesame-Ginger Salmon in Parchment

Continue with the new recipes for the remaining weeks, adjusting based on your preferences and dietary needs. Enjoy the diverse and delicious flavors of the Mediterranean diet!

About the Author

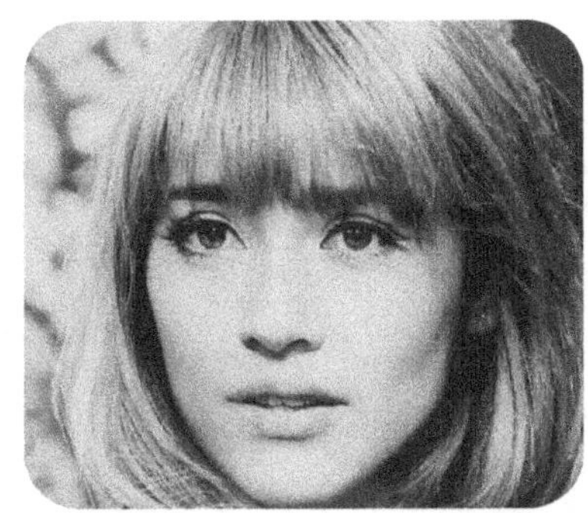

Discover Janie Stafford, a master of crafting flavorful and nutritious recipes that redefine the concept of vibrant living. Janie's passion for food has been nurtured since her early days in the kitchen, and has since taken her to many different countries, where she has been inspired by a variety of culinary traditions. Janie is more than just a chef; she is a dedicated advocate for healthy living. Her exploration into the science of nutrition has become the foundation of her culinary philosophy, which seamlessly combines taste and nourishment in every dish she creates. Janie is an expert in creating recipes that bring out the vibrant flavors of fresh, whole ingredients.

Her dishes demonstrate that food can be both indulgent and healthy, a celebration of nourishment for both body and soul. Janie believes that healthy living is not a chore, but a celebration. Every meal is an opportunity for joy, and every ingredient has a story to tell.

Through her recipes, she invites you to savor the joys of a balanced and delicious life. Whether you are an experienced home cook or just beginning your culinary journey, Janie Stafford invites you to join her on this flavorful journey. Explore the world of Janie Stafford, where the love of cooking meets the art of healthy, delicious living.

Book Content

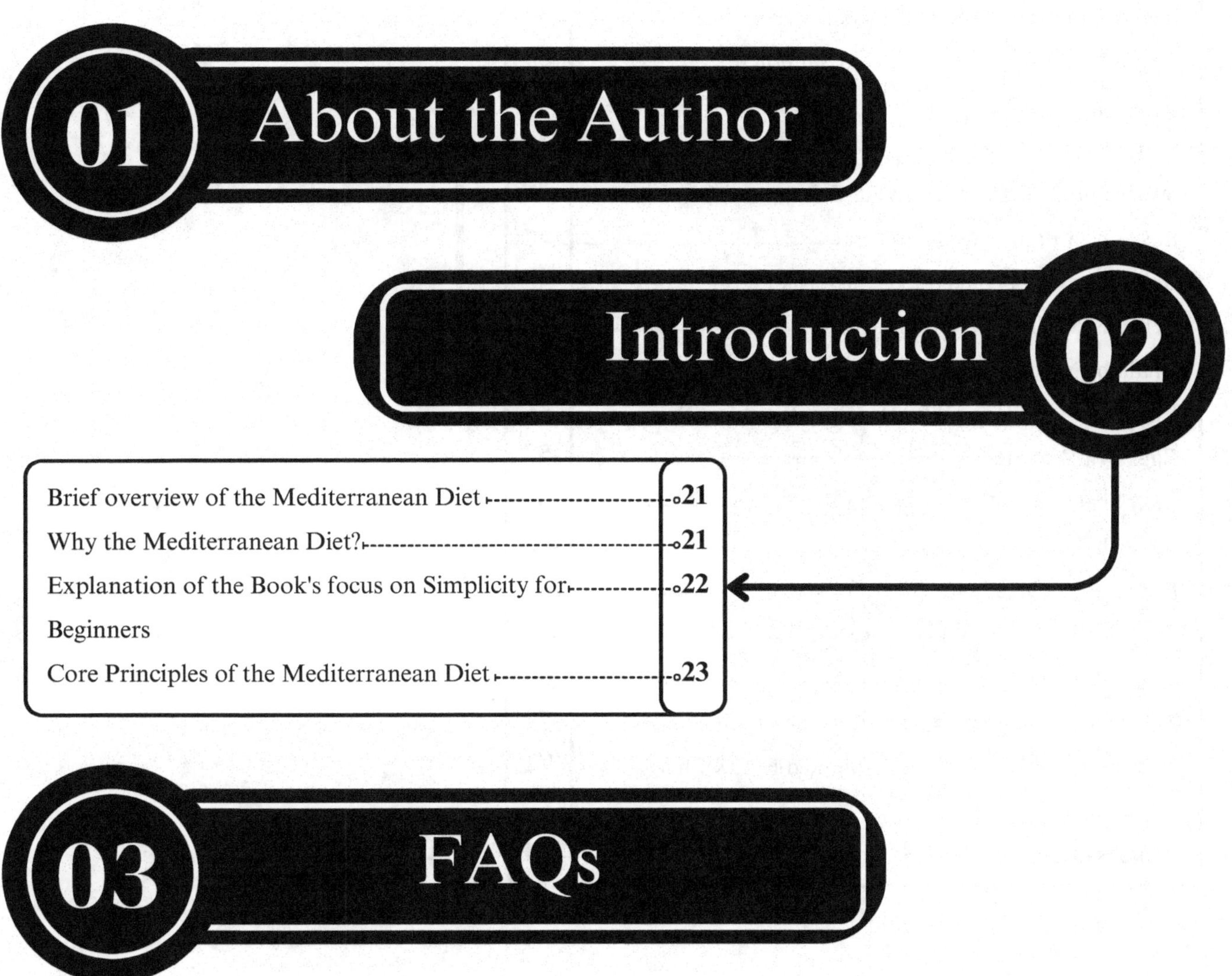

01 About the Author

Introduction **02**

03 FAQs

Breakfast 04

05 Lunch

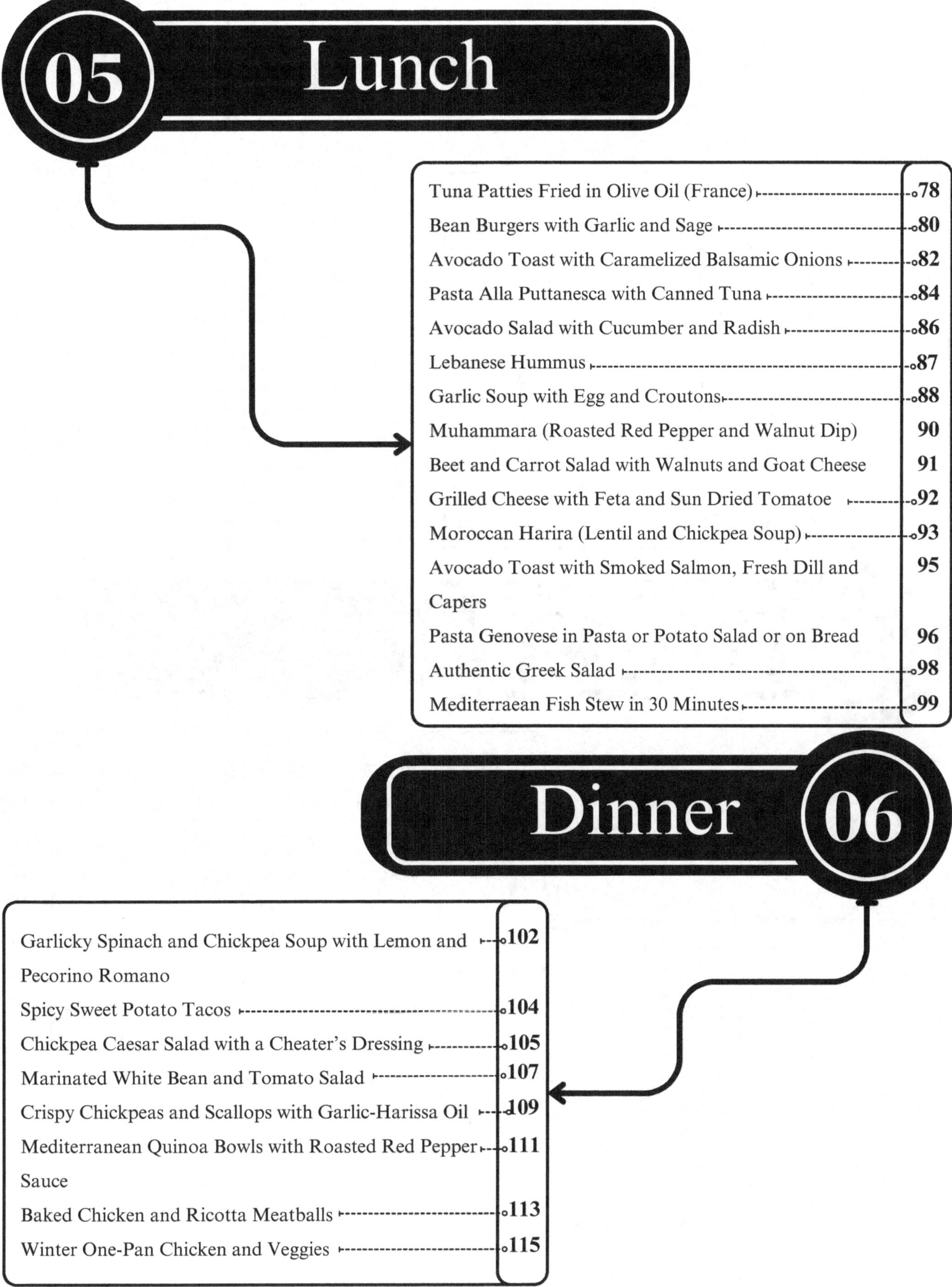

Dinner 06

07 Beans, Grains and Pasta

Fish and Seafood 08

09 Fruits and Snacks

Poultry and Meat 10

11 Sides, Salads and Soup

Vegetable Mains and Meatless Recipes — 12

13 — Desserts

Conclusion 14

15 I have a Request

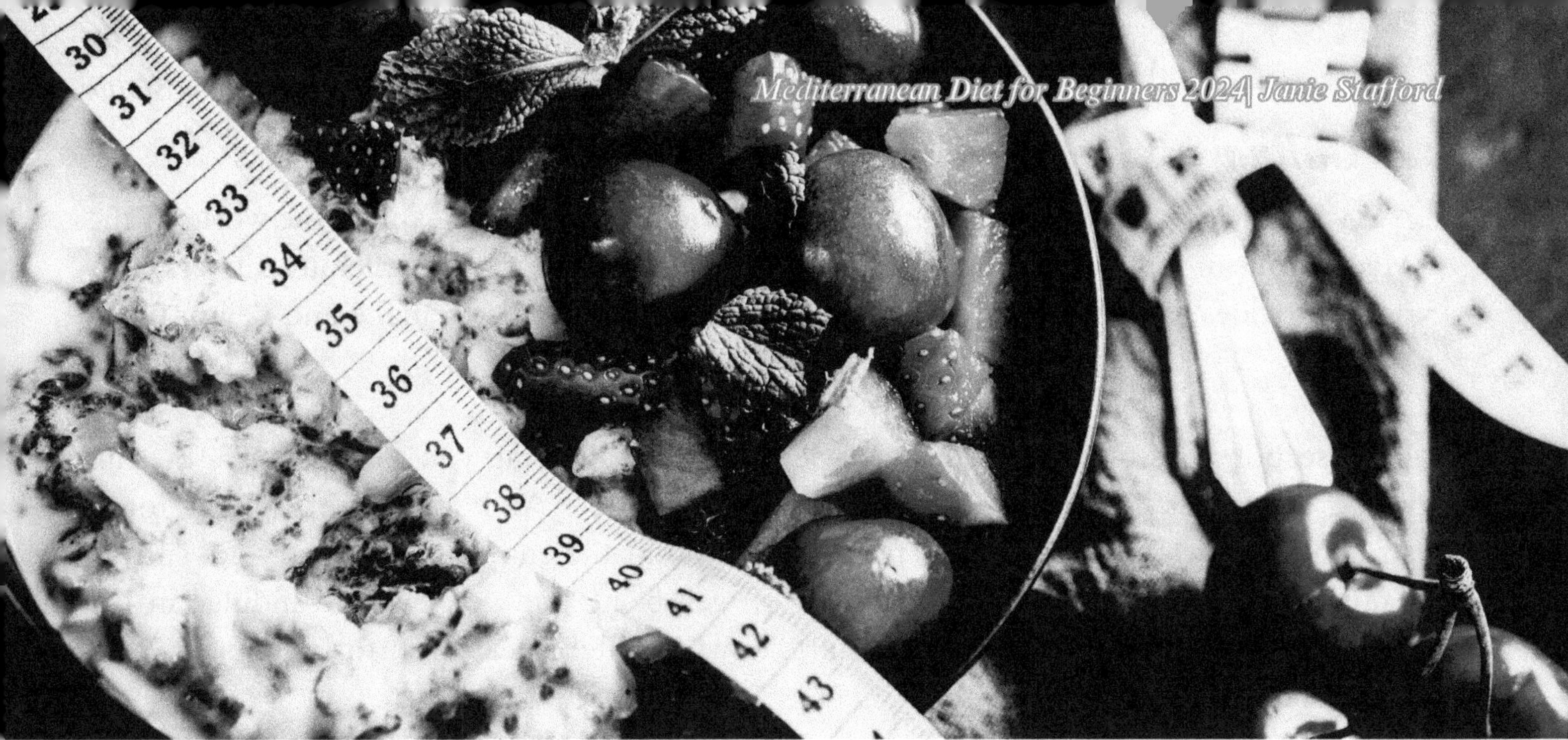

Introduction

Brief overview of the Mediterranean diet

Welcome to "Mediterranean Diet for Beginners 2024"! Starting a journey to a healthier lifestyle has never been easier or more inviting. This book is designed for those just beginning, introducing you to the scrumptious and heart-healthy Mediterranean diet.

The Mediterranean diet is not just a collection of recipes; it is a lifestyle that is praised for its straightforwardness, freshness, and deliciousness. In the following pages, we will uncover the mysteries of this renowned diet, making it easier to understand for those just beginning their culinary journey.

Why the Mediterranean Diet?

One may ask, "What makes the Mediterranean diet so special?" The answer is simple: its demonstrated health advantages and the delight of relishing meals inspired by the sunny coasts of the Mediterranean. This diet is not about limitations, but rather a celebration of healthy, nutrientpacked foods that nurture both the body and spirit.

A Culinary Adventure Awaits: Recipes and Meal Plans

Are you ready to embark on a journey of health and flavor? Let's explore the world of the Mediterranean diet for beginners. From energizing breakfasts to delicious dinners, this book provides a wide selection of recipes that are both simple to make and delightful to enjoy.

Each section focuses on a particular type of cuisine, allowing you to experience the full range of flavors the Mediterranean diet has to offer. And for those looking for a structured start, our 28-day meal plan awaits you at the end of this culinary adventure. Transform your meals into a celebration of well-being and get ready to indulge in the Mediterranean lifestyle. The journey starts now! Mediterranean Diet for Beginners 2024| Janie Stafford

Explanation of the book's focus on simplicity for beginners

Embarking on a new dietary journey can be both exciting and daunting, particularly for those taking their first steps towards a healthier lifestyle. To make this journey easier, "Mediterranean Diet for Beginners 2024" is designed with a focus on simplicity, so that everyone, especially those new to the Mediterranean diet, can approach it with confidence.

This book provides a guiding light for beginners, breaking down the core principles of the Mediterranean diet into easy-to-understand concepts. It also celebrates wholesome and readily available ingredients, curating recipes that highlight the natural flavors of fresh fruits, vegetables, whole grains, and lean proteins.

To make the Mediterranean diet accessible to all, regardless of cooking expertise, the recipes are designed with simplicity in mind, featuring easy-to-follow instructions and minimal cooking times

The journey towards a healthier lifestyle is most successful when it involves sustainable habits. By promoting simplicity, we encourage the formation of long-lasting dietary choices that can seamlessly integrate into daily life. To accommodate different palates, the book provides a diverse range of recipes, so that everyone can find something to suit their taste.

Simplicity should not be mistaken for monotony. Instead, it serves as a gateway to culinary exploration. By making the Mediterranean diet approachable, we invite beginners to experiment with new flavors, textures, and ingredients, fostering a sense of curiosity and enjoyment in the kitchen.

Core Principles of the Mediterranean diet

The Mediterranean diet isn't just a set of rules to follow, but rather a way of life that focuses on healthy eating and shared culinary traditions. Here are the core principles

Emphasis on plant-based foods: Make sure to include plenty of fruits and vegetables in your diet, aiming for at least 5 servings daily and varying the colors and types. Whole grains are preferable to refined grains, so opt for brown rice, quinoa, oats, whole-wheat bread, and pasta.

Legumes and beans, such as lentils, chickpeas, beans, and peas, should be included several times a week for protein and fiber. Nuts and seeds are also great for healthy fats, fiber, and protein, so enjoy a handful daily

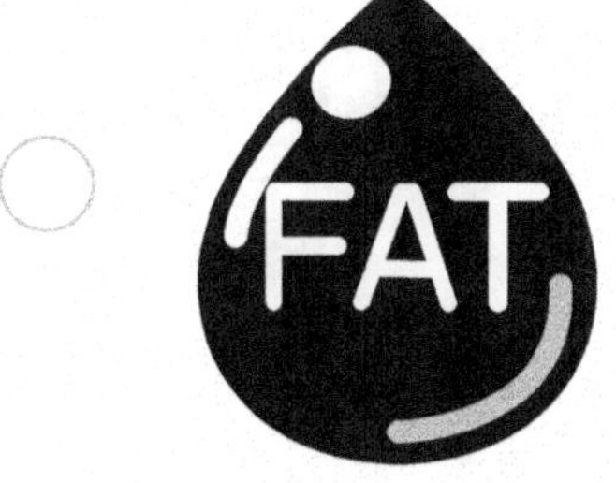

Healthy fats: Olive oil should be your primary source of fat, so use it for cooking and drizzle it on salads. You can also have moderate portions of other healthy fats, such as avocados, fatty fish like salmon and tuna, and nuts.

Balance and moderation: Red meat should be consumed sparingly, opting for lean cuts and prioritizing poultry and fish instead. Dairy products should be enjoyed in moderation for calcium and probiotics. Processed foods, sugary drinks, and unhealthy fats should be avoided.

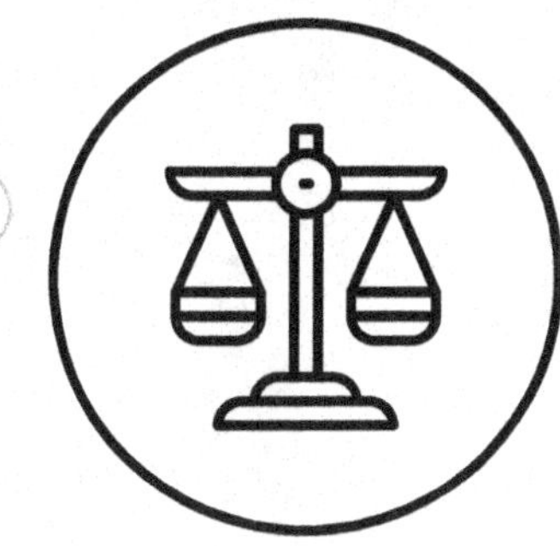

Lifestyle elements: Mindful eating is important, so savor your food, eat slowly, and pay attention to hunger and satiety cues. Regular physical activity is also essential, so aim for at least 30 minutes of moderate-intensity exercise most days of the week.

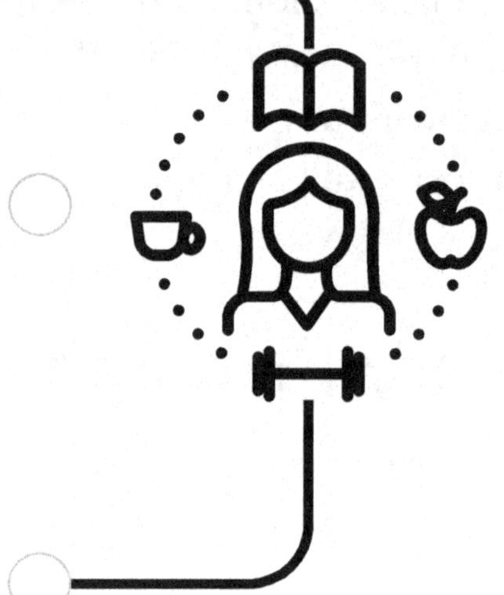

Social connection is also important, so enjoy meals with friends and family, fostering a sense of community and appreciating the social aspect of food. Sustainability is also key, so choose seasonal and local ingredients whenever possible, supporting your community and minimizing environmental impact.

Remember: The Mediterranean diet is a flexible approach, not a rigid one, so adapt it to your individual needs and preferences. Enjoyment and pleasure are central to the diet, so choose delicious and satisfying foods that you look forward to eating. Consistency is key, so focus on incorporating these principles into your daily life for long-term health benefits.

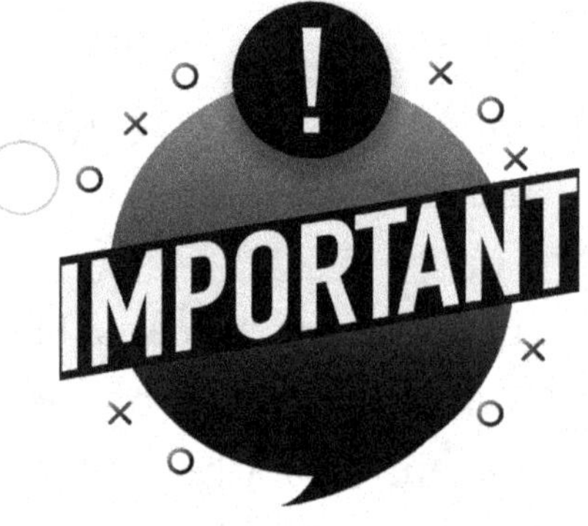

Frequently Asked questions 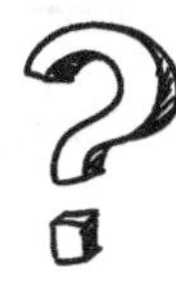

Can I lose weight on this diet?

Can a vegan follow this diet?

Are there any gluten-free options?

Can a diabetic patient follow the Mediterranean diet?

Is this diet suitable for the whole family?

Do I have to drink alcohol?

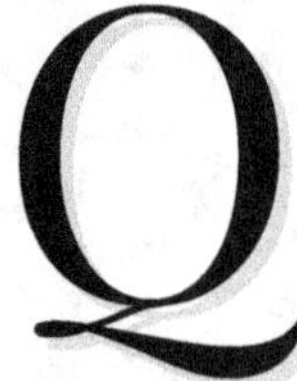
Can I lose weight on this diet?

Definitely! The Mediterranean diet is not about depriving yourself or cutting out food groups. It encourages whole, unprocessed foods, which gives you lots of options and makes it easier to keep up with in the long run. This is essential for successful, lasting weight loss.

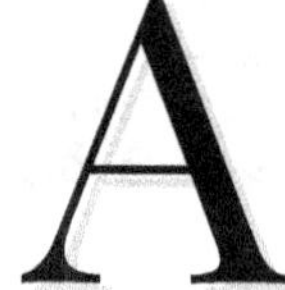

Can a vegan follow this diet?

Yes, it is possible to modify the Mediterranean diet to fit a vegan lifestyle. Vegans can not only follow the Mediterranean diet, but they can also enjoy a healthy and tasty version of it, known as the vegan Mediterranean diet for beginners 2024.

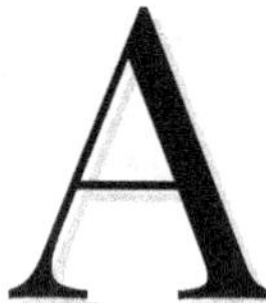

Can a diabetic patient follow the Mediterranean diet?

Yes, the Mediterranean diet is often suggested for people with diabetes because of its focus on whole, nutrient-rich foods and its potential to help manage blood sugar levels. This diet encourages whole grains, fruits, and vegetables with a low glycemic index, which means they release sugar into the bloodstream more gradually, avoiding sudden increases.

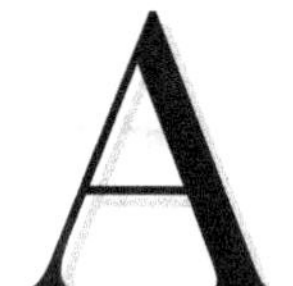

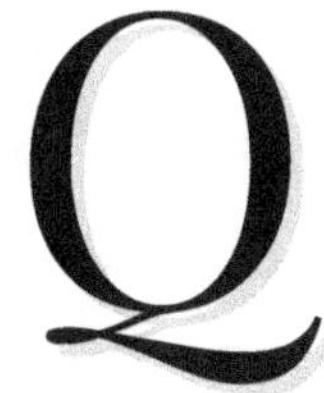

Are there any gluten-free options?

Definitely! The Mediterranean diet has lots of naturally gluten-free options, making it a great choice for people with gluten sensitivity or celiac disease

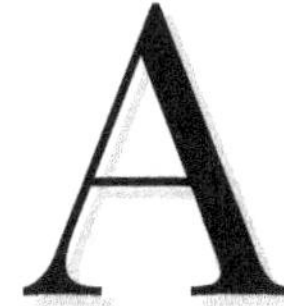

Is this diet suitable for the whole family?

Absolutely! The Mediterranean diet is often seen as a great option for the entire family. It emphasizes a wide range of fresh and delicious foods, making it easy to adjust to different tastes and dietary requirements.

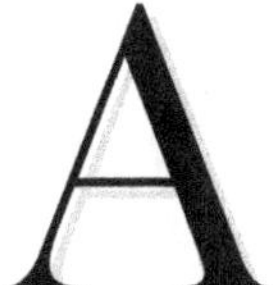

Do I have to drink alcohol?

No need to worry if you don't want to drink alcohol to follow the Mediterranean diet. It's not a must-have component of the diet, even though it's often associated with it. The main focus of the Mediterranean diet is to have a balanced and varied intake of nutrient-rich foods. So, if you don't want to include alcoholic beverages for any reason, you can still enjoy the benefits of the Mediterranean diet.

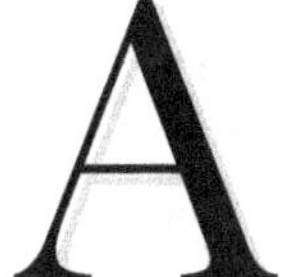

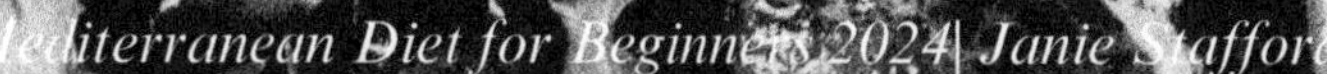

BREAKFAST

◆——◆

RECIPES

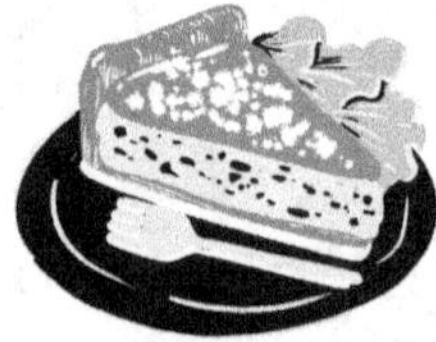

Crustless Quiche With Spinach And Mushrooms

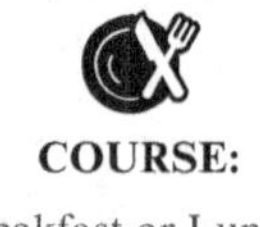

PREP TIME:	**COOK TIME:**	**SERVINGS:**	**COURSE:**
20 mins	35 mins	8	Breakfast or Lunch

Nutritional Value:	Calories: 143.9kcal	fat: 9.9g	carb:4.7g	Protein: 9.4g

INGREDIENTS:

- 5 eggs
- 1 cup whole milk
- 4 ounces Fontina cheese or mozzarella
- 1 tablespoon extra virgin olive oil, plus more for the pan
- 8 ounces sliced mushrooms
- ½ medium yellow onion, minced
- 3 large cloves garlic, minced
- 1 teaspoon dried thyme
- 1 teaspoon kosher salt
- ½ teaspoon black pepper
- 1 ½ tablespoons balsamic vinegar
- 2 cups packed baby spinach leaves

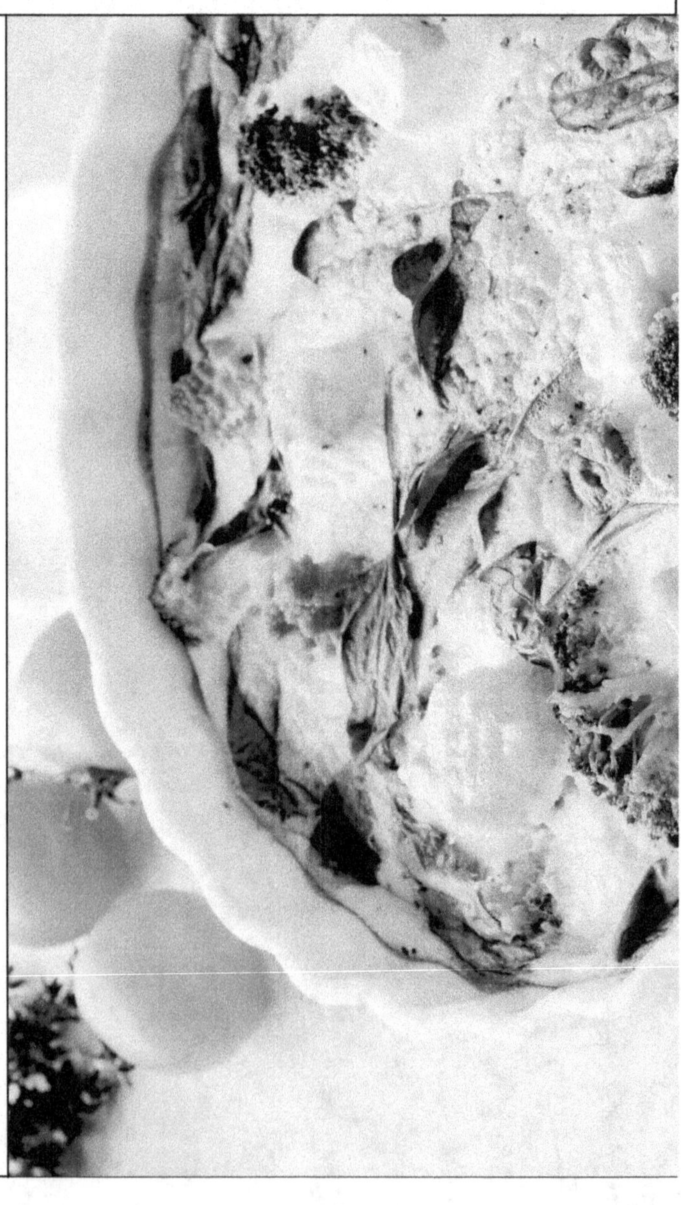

DIRECTIONS:

- Preheat the oven and prepare the pan: Preheat the oven to 375°F and lightly coat a 9-inch pie plate with olive oil. Place it on a baking sheet.

- Whisk the eggs and cube the cheese: In a bowl, vigorously whisk together the eggs and milk. Cut the Fontina cheese into cubes and set aside.

- Prepare the vegetables: Heat a large skillet over medium-high heat and add the olive oil. When it starts to shimmer, add the mushrooms, onion, and garlic. Sprinkle with thyme, salt, and pepper. Cook until the mushrooms shrink and the onions become translucent, which should take around 10 to 15 minutes depending on the size of the mushrooms. Drizzle the balsamic vinegar over the vegetables and stir, cooking for another minute or two. Add the spinach, stirring until it wilts, which should take about 3 minutes. Taste and adjust the seasoning to your preference.

- Combine: Place the cooked vegetables into the pie plate, sprinkle with the cubed cheese, and pour the egg mixture over the top. Make sure it is full up to the rim. Carefully move the baking sheet to the oven.

- Bake: Set the timer for 35 minutes and bake until the center is set. Allow the dish to cool at room temperature for about 10 minutes before serving

Spanakopita Egg Muffins (Easy Egg Bite Recipe!)

 **PREP TIME:** 5 mins	 **COOK TIME:** 25 mins	 **SERVINGS:** 6	 **COURSE:** Breakfast or Lunch

Nutritional Value:	Calories: 138.9kcal	Fat: 8.5g	Carb:4.7g	Protein: 11.6g

INGREDIENTS:

- Extra virgin olive oil
- 12 large eggs
- 1 ½ teaspoons dried oregano
- ¾ teaspoon ground black pepper
- ¾ teaspoon sweet paprika
- ¼ teaspoon baking powder
- Kosher salt
- 1 9-ounce package frozen chopped spinach, thawed and completely drained (wring out any water)
- ¾ small yellow onion finely chopped (about ¾ cup)
- 1 ¼ cup roughly chopped parsley leaves and tender stems
- ¼ cup chopped mint leaves
- 4 large garlic cloves minced
- 1 6-ounce block feta cheese, crumbled (about 1 cup)

DIRECTIONS:

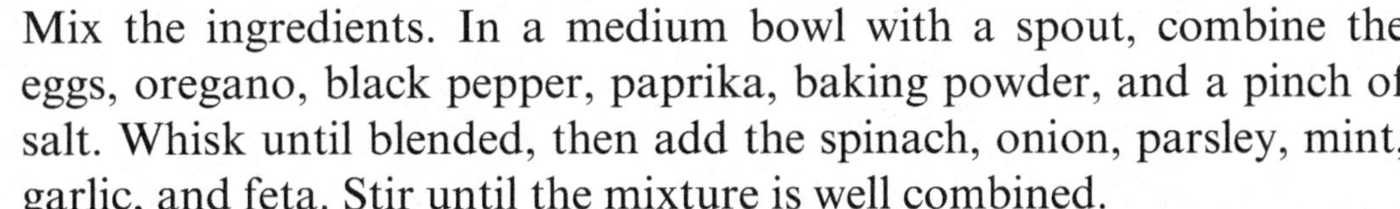

Prepare the oven. Place a rack in the center of the oven and preheat to 350°F. Generously brush the bottom and sides of a muffin tin with olive oil.

Mix the ingredients. In a medium bowl with a spout, combine the eggs, oregano, black pepper, paprika, baking powder, and a pinch of salt. Whisk until blended, then add the spinach, onion, parsley, mint, garlic, and feta. Stir until the mixture is well combined.

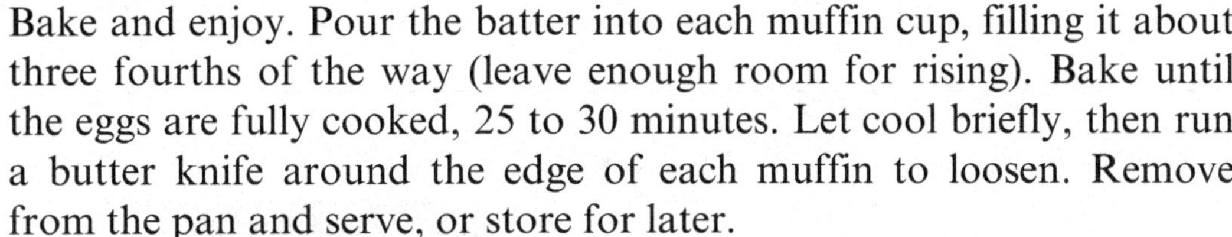

Bake and enjoy. Pour the batter into each muffin cup, filling it about three fourths of the way (leave enough room for rising). Bake until the eggs are fully cooked, 25 to 30 minutes. Let cool briefly, then run a butter knife around the edge of each muffin to loosen. Remove from the pan and serve, or store for later.

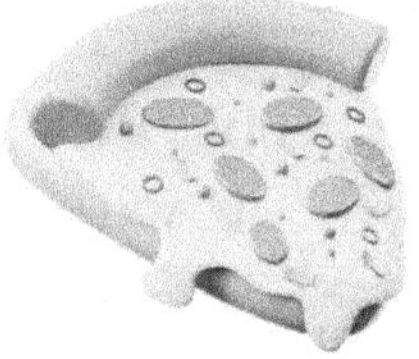 Pita Breakfast Pizza with Za'atar

 **PREP TIME:** 5 mins	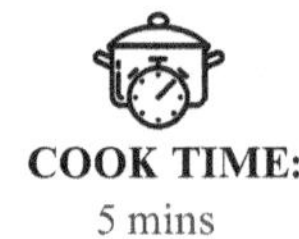 **COOK TIME:** 5 mins	 **SERVINGS:** 8 slices	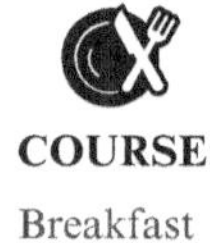 **COURSE:** Breakfast

Nutritional Value:	Calories: 83.6kcal	Fat: 4.1g	Carb:6.8g	Protein: 5.3g

INGREDIENTS:

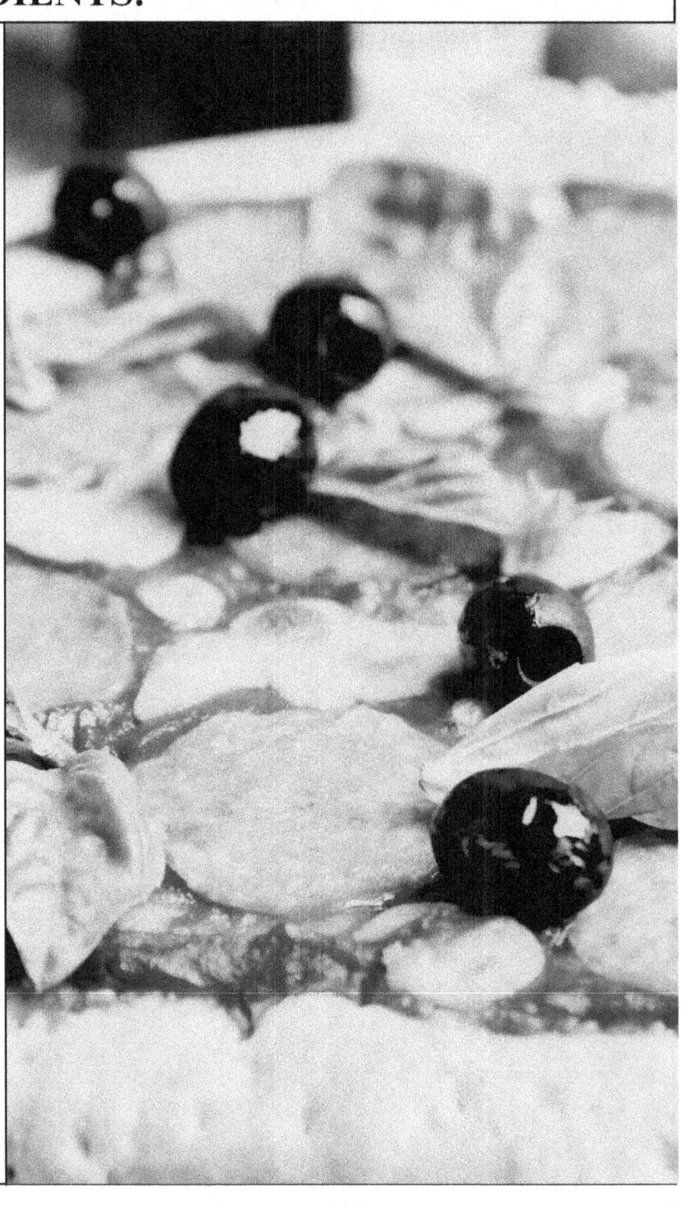

- 1 large whole wheat pita bread or 2 medium pitas (or your favorite flatbread)
- Extra-virgin olive oil
- ½ cup grated mozzarella, more to your liking
- 1 teaspoon za'atar, more to your liking
- Pinch red pepper flakes (optional)
- 1 shallot, thinly sliced into rounds
- 1 Roma tomato or a handful of cherry tomatoes, sliced
- 2 hard boiled eggs, peeled and grated or chopped
- Kosher salt

DIRECTIONS:

- Preheat the oven: Preheat the oven to 375°F with a rack in the center

- Place the pita (or flatbread) on a baking sheet and brush the top with olive oil.

- Sprinkle the mozzarella, za'atar, and red pepper flakes on top of the pita. On top, scatter the shallots, tomatoes, and grated egg. Season with kosher salt to taste.

- Bake for 5 minutes, or until the cheese has melted and the pita is somewhat crunchy

- Finish with a last sprinkle of za'atar if desired. Eat it while it's still hot!

NOTES:

- Because the eggs are grated, they should be fully cooked but not overcooked. See our favorite way in our How To Boil Eggs guide. If you don't have a cheese grater, just roughly cut the eggs with a knife.

- For the finest flavor, choose a low moisture whole milk mozzarella. A milky, creamy mozzarella is fantastic in a caprese salad, but it gets soggy as it melts.

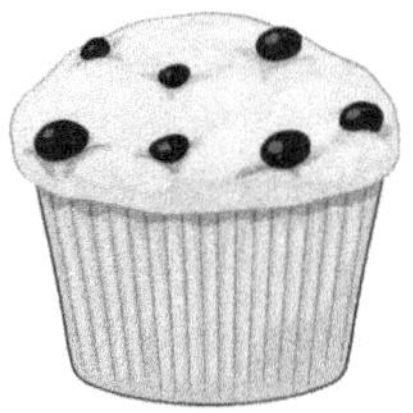

Healthy Blueberry Muffins (Whole Wheat!)

PREP TIME:
10 mins

COOK TIME:
22 mins

SERVINGS:
12 muffins

COURSE:
Breakfast, Dessert or Snack

Nutritional Value:	Calories: 178.6kcal	Fat: 6.9g	Carb: 28.2g	Protein: 3.2g

INGREDIENTS:

- ¾ cups (210g) white whole wheat flour
- 1 teaspoon baking powder
- ½ teaspoon baking soda
- ½ teaspoon kosher salt
- ¼ teaspoon ground cinnamon
- ½ cup honey
- ½ cup unsweetened apple sauce
- ⅓ cup olive oil, plus more for coating the tray
- ¼ cup milk
- 1 large egg
- 1 teaspoon vanilla extract
- 1 ½ cups fresh or frozen blueberries

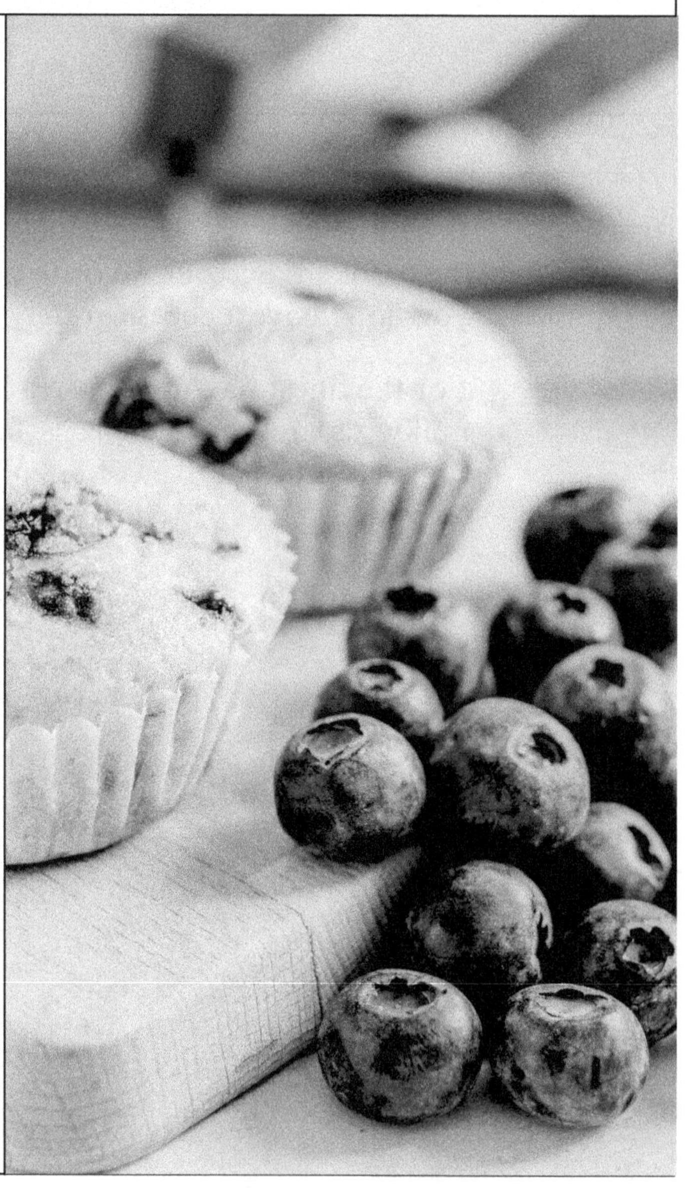

DIRECTIONS:

Prepare yourself: Preheat the oven to 375 degrees Fahrenheit. Grease a regular 12-cup muffin pan lightly or line with muffin liners.

In a large mixing basin, whisk together the flour, baking powder, baking soda, salt, and cinnamon.

In a medium mixing bowl, blend the honey, apple sauce, olive oil, milk, egg, and vanilla extract until well incorporated.

Pour the wet ingredients into the dry ingredients and mix together with a spatula until barely incorporated. Avoid overmixing. It's fine if there are some lumps.

Toss in the blueberries: With a spatula, scatter the blueberries throughout the batter.

Scoop or pour the batter into the prepared muffin tin, dividing it evenly among the wells. Fill each well to about 34 percent capacity.

Cook the muffins for 22 minutes, or until a toothpick inserted into one of the muffins comes out clean.

• Allow the muffins to cool in the pan for 10 minutes before turning them out onto a wire rack to cool completely. If necessary, run a butter knife around the edge of each muffin to release it from the pan.

Serve at room temperature or heated. The muffins can be stored at room temperature in an airtight container for up to 4 days.

NOTES:

If you don't have white whole wheat flour, use wcup whole wheat flour mixed with 34 cup allpurpose flour as a substitute.

When you mix muffin batter, you activate the gluten, which enables it to grow and become more elastic. Mix just until the ingredients are mixed. Overactive gluten does not rise, resulting in rough, dense, and dry muffins.

The muffins can be stored at room temperature in an airtight container for up to 4 days. They can also be frozen for up to 3 months in a freezer-safe container or freezer bag. Place frozen muffins on the counter to thaw.

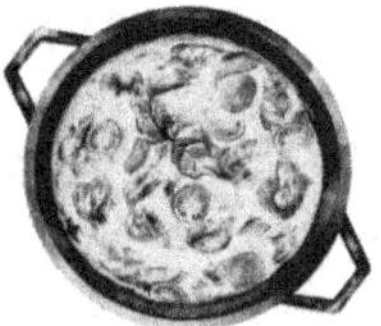

Egg White Frittata with Smoked Salmon

 **PREP TIME:** 15 mins	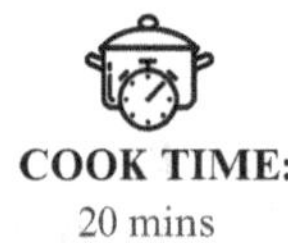 **COOK TIME:** 20 mins	 **SERVINGS:** 8	 **COURSE:** Breakfast, Dessert or Snack

Nutritional Value:	Calories: 104.3kcal	Fat: 5.8g	Carb: 1.1g	Protein: 11.5g

INGREDIENTS:

- 1 tablespoon extra-virgin olive oil
- ½ medium red onion, diced
- 12 large egg whites (about 360g)
- 6 ounces smoked salmon, torn or sliced into bite-size pieces
- 4 ounces soft goat cheese, crumbled
- 1 tablespoon capers, drained and roughly chopped
- 2 tablespoons chopped dill, plus more for garnish
- ¼ teaspoon freshly ground black pepper

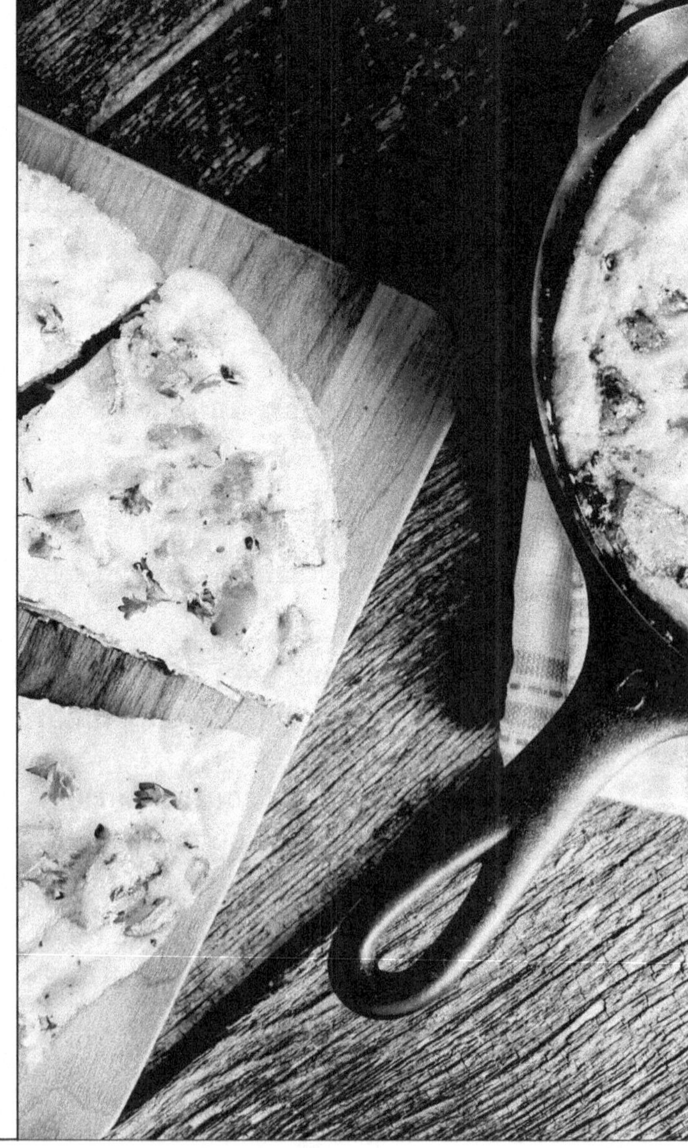

DIRECTIONS:

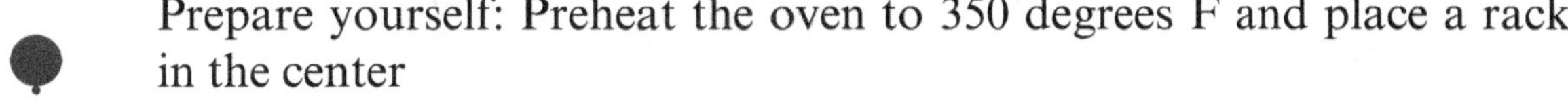

Prepare yourself: Preheat the oven to 350 degrees F and place a rack in the center

In a 10-inch oven-safe nonstick skillet over medium heat, heat the oil. Cook for 3 to 4 minutes, stirring periodically, with the diced onion. The onions should soften, start to brown around the edges, and smell delicious.

While the onions are frying, combine the egg whites in a large mixing dish. Whisk for 30 seconds, or until foamy. Combine the salmon, goat cheese, capers, dill, and black pepper in a mixing bowl.

When the onions have softened, add the egg and salmon combination to the pan. Cook, stirring occasionally, for 3 to 4 minutes, or until the edges begin to firm.

Bake the eggs: Put the pan in the oven for 12 minutes, or until the frittata is set. The frittata should have puffed slightly and be solid in the center.

Allow it cool for a few minutes before slicing into 8 pieces to serve. Garnish with fresh dill before serving.

NOTES:

Frittata can be stored in the fridge for 3-4 days. Allow leftovers to cool to room temperature before storing. Refrigerate in an airtight container or wrapped tightly in plastic

To determine whether your frittata is done, do the "jiggle test." If the middle of the frittata jiggles when you shake the skillet, it needs to cook longer.

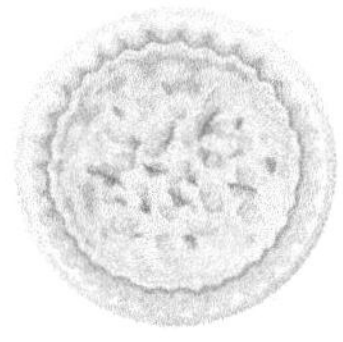

Asparagus Quiche

 PREP TIME: 1hr	 COOK TIME: 35 mins	 SERVINGS: 8	 COURSE: Breakfast, Brunch, Dinner or Lunch

Nutritional Value:	Calories: 229kcal	Fat: 12.1g	Carb: 21.4g	Protein: 9.8g

INGREDIENTS:

For The Dough:

- ¾ cup 90 g all-purpose flour, plus more for dusting
- ¾ cup (85g) whole wheat flour
- ½ teaspoon kosher salt
- ¼ cup extra virgin olive oil
- ¼ cup water

For The Filling:

- 1 teaspoon extra virgin olive oil
- ½ onion thinly sliced
- 12 ounces asparagus, cut into 1-inch pieces
- 1 garlic clove, minced
- ½ cup grated Asiago cheese (56g)
- 4 large eggs
- 1 cup 2% milk
- 1 tablespoon Dijon mustard
- 1 teaspoon chopped fresh thyme or tarragon leaves (optional)
- ½ teaspoon kosher salt, divided
- ⅛ teaspoon freshly ground black pepper

DIRECTIONS:

- Prepare the dough: In a food processor, combine the all-purpose flour, whole wheat flour, and salt and pulse a few times to combine. Pour in the olive oil and pulse until it's dispersed evenly throughout the flour. Add the water and pulse until the mixture clumps and becomes uniformly wet.

- Knead the dough: Place the dough on a lightly floured work area and knead it by hand until it forms a ball. Form the dough into a 1 inch thick disk. Wrap the disk in plastic and let it aside for 1 hour at room temperature. This interval of rest allows the flour to hydrate and the gluten to relax.

- Prepare to bake: Preheat the oven to 375°F with a rack in the center. Flour lightly dust your countertop. Roll out the dough to an 11-inch circle, approximately 18-inch thick, with a floured rolling pin.

- Transfer the dough: Carefully roll the dough around the rolling pin before unrolling it into a 9-inch pie dish. To line the pie dish, gently press the dough in. Roll and fold the overhang of dough to form the edges of the pie dish, removing excess dough as you go around the circumference. Crimp the edges with your fingers or a fork, or leave them alone for a more rustic look.

- Cover the crust with parchment paper or tin foil and bake it blind. Bake for 20 minutes with pie weights or dried beans. Bake for 10 minutes after removing the parchment and pie weights.

- While the crust is baking, heat 1 teaspoon olive oil in a large nonstick skillet over medium heat. Cook, turning periodically with a wooden spoon, until the onions are transparent and softened, about 5 minutes. Cook until the asparagus is tender and brilliant green, about 5 minutes more. Cook for 1 minute, or until the garlic is aromatic. Remove the vegetables from the heat and place them in the blind-baked crust. Garnish with shredded cheese.

- To make the egg filling, whisk together the eggs, milk, Dijon mustard, herbs (if using), 12 teaspoon salt, and 18 teaspoon pepper in a large mixing dish. Fill the crust 14 inch from the top with the egg mixture. Depending on the depth of your pie pan, you may not use all of it.

- Bake, chill, slice, and serve the quiche for 30-35 minutes, or until the edges are set but the center jiggles slightly.Allow the quiche to cool for at least 15 minutes before slicing and serving. Serve hot, cold, or at room temperature.

NOTES:

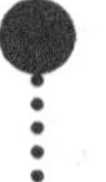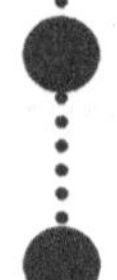

As the crust blind bakes, make sure you have something to weigh it with, such as dried beans, grains, pie weights, or clean pennies.

Hold the bottom of the stalk with one hand and the middle with the other to trim the asparagus. Bend it until it snaps (the delicate and woody parts will naturally snap together).

Soft Scrambled Eggs

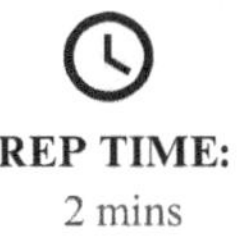

PREP TIME:
2 mins

COOK TIME:
8 mins

SERVINGS:
2

COURSE:
Breakfast

Nutritional Value:	Calories: 206.2kcal	Fat: 16.4g	Carb: 1.2g	Protein: 12.7g

INGREDIENTS:

- 4 large eggs
- Kosher salt
- Extra virgin olive oil
- 2 to 3 tablespoons Greek yogurt
- 1 tablespoon chopped chives

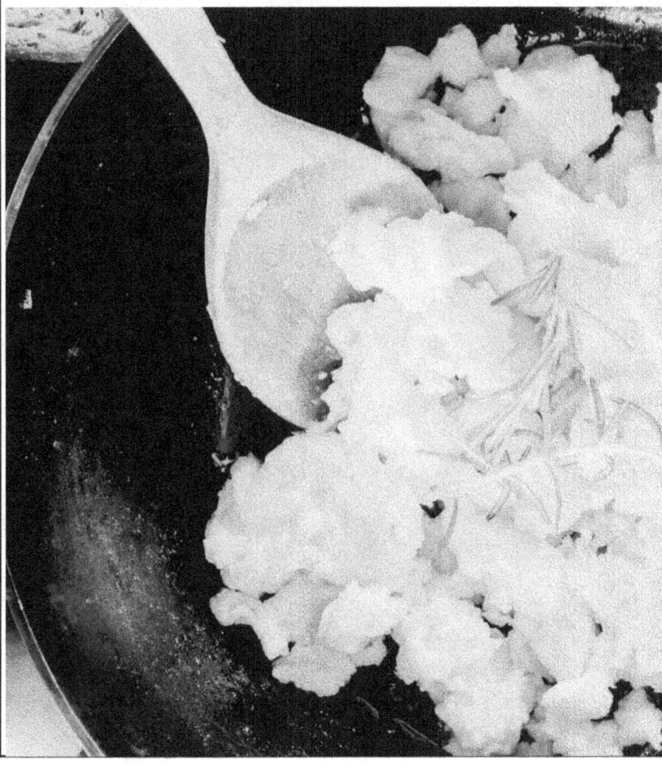

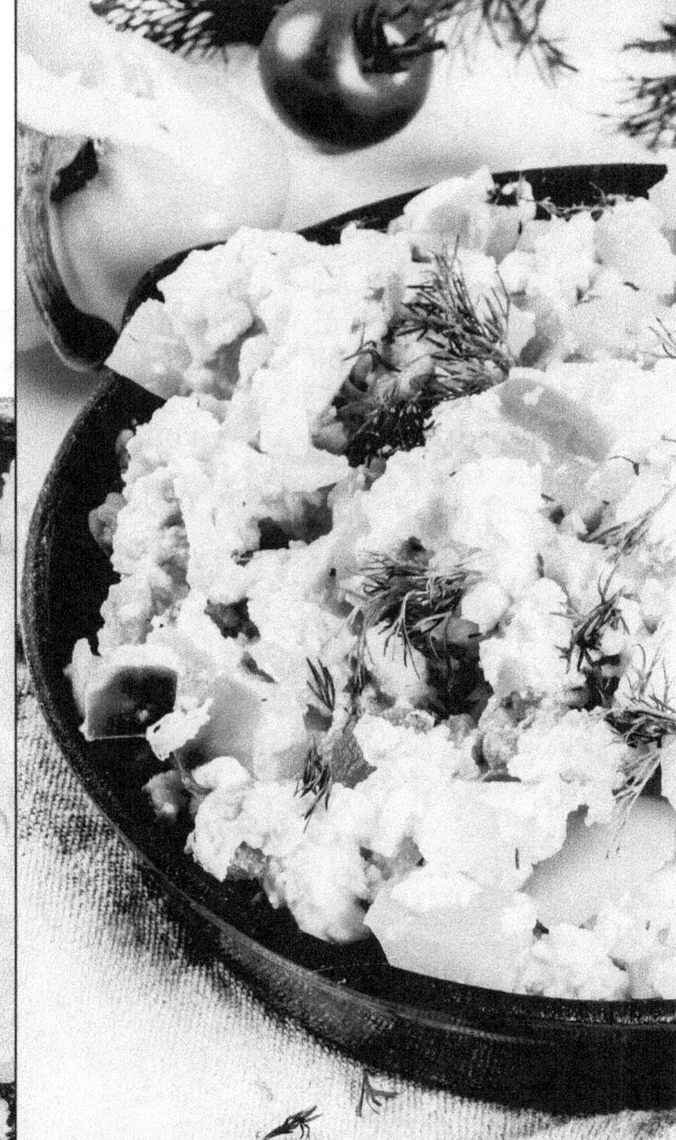

DIRECTIONS:

- Prepare the eggs: Place the eggs in a small mixing bowl and season generously with kosher salt. Whisk in 1 teaspoon olive oil until blended.

- Oil the skillet: Heat 1-2 tablespoons olive oil in a small nonstick skillet over medium heat. Warm the olive oil for about 30 seconds before adding the whisked eggs.

- Cook the eggs: Cook the eggs over medium heat, turning often with a rubber spatula, until the eggs begin to set (some moist areas are good).

- Remove from the heat and stir in the Greek yogurt. Stir until the yogurt is completely blended and the eggs are completely set. Season with salt and pepper to taste.

- Transfer the scrambled eggs to serving plates and top with chives. Enjoy right away.

NOTES:

- Warm both the pan and the eggs at the same time, stirring frequently. Starting the eggs on a hot pan will cause them to dry out.

- To avoid scraping your nonstick pan, use a rubber spatula.

- Because residual heat will cause your eggs to continue to cook, turn off the fire and whisk in the Greek yogurt just before the eggs are entirely cooked.

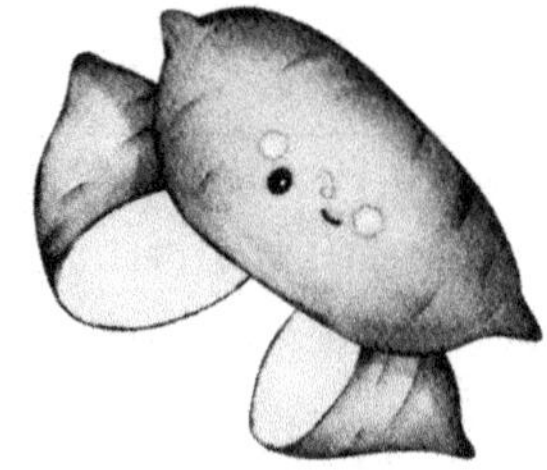

Sweet Potato Hash Recipe with Za'atar and Chickpeas

 **PREP TIME:** 10 mins	 **COOK TIME:** 20 mins	 **SERVINGS:** 4	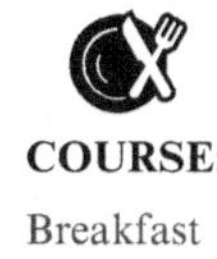 **COURSE:** Breakfast

Nutritional Value:	Calories: 317kcal	Fat: 15.9g	Carb: 34.8g	Protein: 10.3g

INGREDIENTS:

- 3 tablespoons extra-virgin olive oil
- 1 medium red onion, chopped
- 2 small sweet potatoes, about 1 ½ pounds total, peeled and cut into ½-inch cubes
- 1 cup canned chickpeas, drained and rinsed
- Kosher salt and ground black pepper
- 1 teaspoon ground coriander
- ½ teaspoon ground cumin
- ½ teaspoon sweet paprika
- ½ teaspoon ground turmeric
- 2 large garlic cloves, minced
- 1 large red bell pepper, cored, seeded and chopped
- 1 tablespoon za'atar, plus more as desired
- 1 teaspoon distilled white vinegar
- 4 large eggs

DIRECTIONS:

Heat the olive oil in a 12-inch cast-iron skillet over medium-high heat until shimmering but not smoking. Combine the red onion, sweet potatoes, and chickpeas in a mixing bowl. Season with a generous amount of salt and black pepper (12 teaspoons each). Combine the coriander, cumin, paprika, and turmeric in a mixing bowl. To blend, stir everything together. Cook, stirring regularly, for 10 to 15 minutes, or until the onion is well caramelized and the sweet potatoes have softened significantly.

Turn the heat down to medium. Combine the garlic and bell pepper in a mixing bowl. Cook, turning regularly, for another 5 to 10 minutes, or until the pepper has softened and the potatoes are cooked through. Garnish with za'atar.

Meanwhile, put a medium pot of water to a medium-low simmer and add the vinegar. Each egg should be broken into a small bowl or ramekin. Gently stir the heating water and delicately insert each egg; the egg whites should wrap around the yolk. Cook for 3 minutes, then remove the eggs with a slotted spoon from the simmering water and place them on a paper towel to drain quickly. Season with salt, pepper, and more za'atar to taste.

Divide the sweet potato hash among four bowls and top with a poached egg in each. Serve right away.

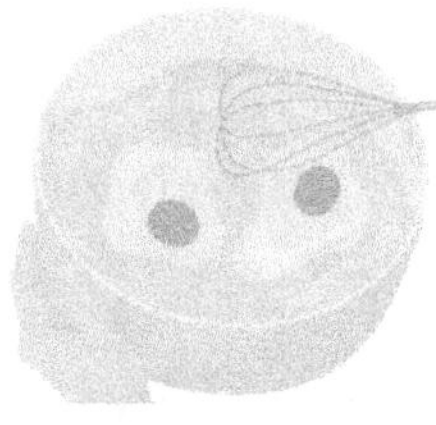

Easy Oven Baked Eggs

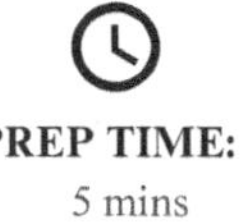 **PREP TIME:** 5 mins	 **COOK TIME:** 8 mins	 **SERVINGS:** 2	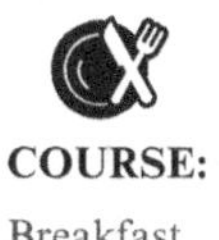 **COURSE:** Breakfast

Nutritional Value:	Calories: 125.8kcal	Fat: 8.4g	Carb: 0.6g	Protein: 11.1g

INGREDIENTS:

- Extra virgin olive oil
- 2 to 4 Large eggs
- Kosher salt and black pepper
- Red pepper flakes or Aleppo pepper, optional
- Optional Toppings:
- Crumbled feta cheese
- Chopped chives
- Chopped parsley
- Microgreens
- Small diced tomatoes

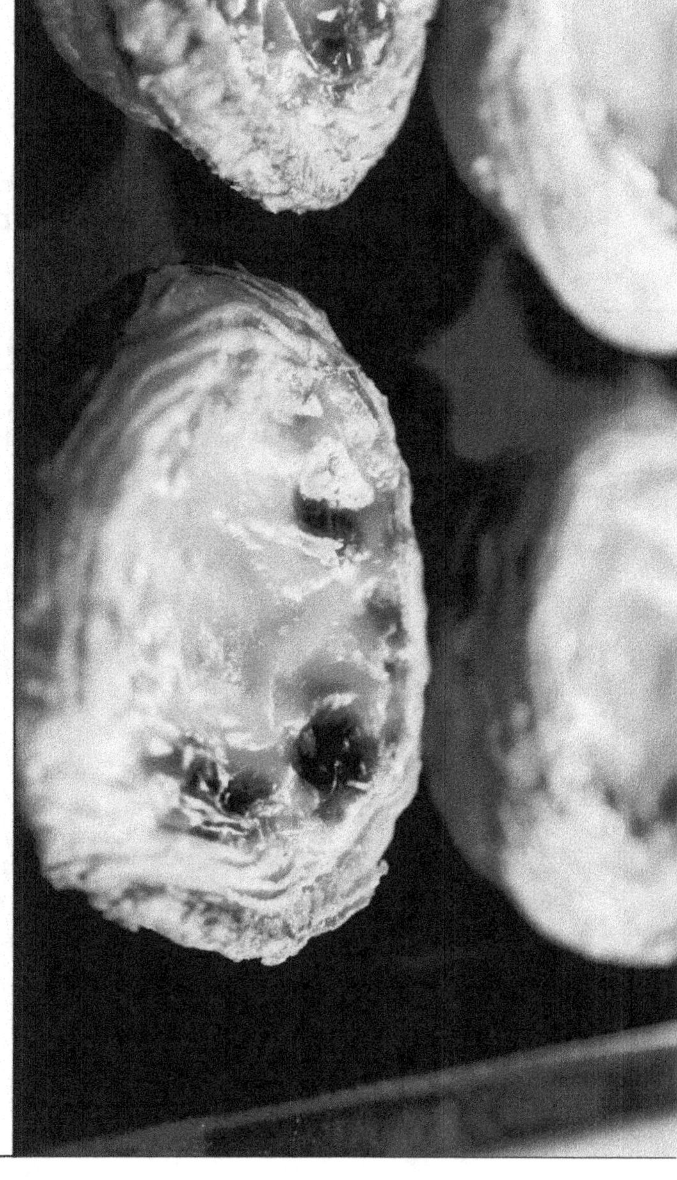

DIRECTIONS:

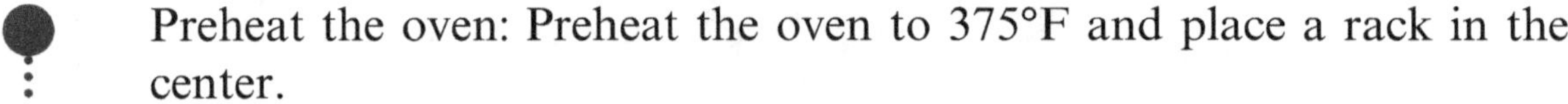
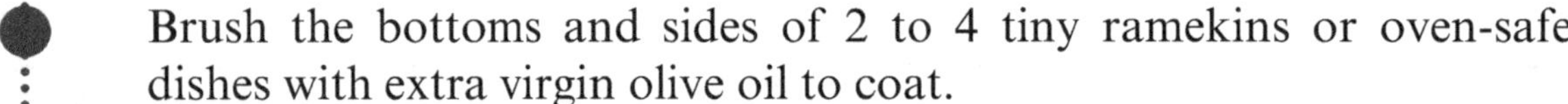

- Preheat the oven: Preheat the oven to 375°F and place a rack in the center.

- Brush the bottoms and sides of 2 to 4 tiny ramekins or oven-safe dishes with extra virgin olive oil to coat.

- Add the egg(s): Crack 1 egg into each dish, depending on size (a 4 12 - inch round ramekin will take 2 eggs).

- Bake: Arrange the ramekins on a sheet pan and place the sheet pan on the hot oven's center rack. Bake for 8 minutes, or until the egg whites are barely set. The yolks should still be fluid, so keep an eye on them to avoid overcooking (remember, the egg whites will continue to set after you remove them from the oven). If you prefer firmer yolks, keep the eggs in the oven for a couple of minutes longer.

- Garnish and serve: Remove the eggs from the oven and season with kosher salt, black pepper, and, if you want a little heat, a dash of red pepper flakes or Aleppo pepper. Garnish with your preferred toppings (feta, fresh herbs, or small diced tomatoes). Serve right away!

NOTES:

- Make it your own: Almost anything goes with eggs! Add a pinch of Aleppo pepper, fresh herbs, and crumbled cheese to taste.

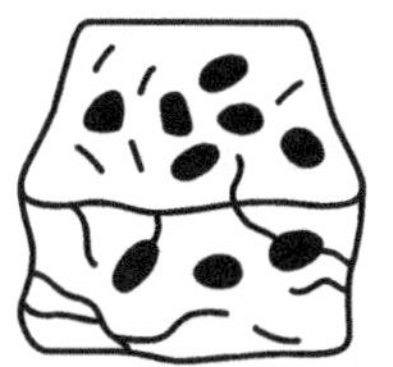

Breakfast Strata (Baked Egg Casserole)

| 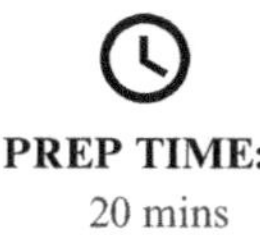
PREP TIME:
20 mins | 
COOK TIME:
1hr | 
SERVINGS:
10 | 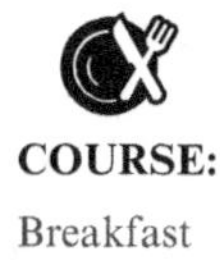
COURSE:
Breakfast |
| --- | --- | --- | --- |

Nutritional Value:	Calories: 337.5kcal	Fat: 16g	Carb: 29.4g	Protein: 19g

INGREDIENTS:

- 2 teaspoons olive oil, plus more for greasing the baking dish
- 3 cups chopped spinach, packed
- 4 cloves garlic, minced
- 1 pound about 6 cups crusty bread, cut into large cubes
- 4 ounces chevre cheese
- 1 cup shredded parmesan cheese
- 3 large roasted red peppers, chopped (about 1 cup)
- 3 ounces prosciutto, torn to bite-size pieces
- 4 scallions or chives, chopped
- 8 eggs
- cups whole milk
- 1 teaspoon Italian seasoning
- 1 teaspoon kosher salt
- ½ teaspoon black pepper

DIRECTIONS:

- Preheat the oven to 350 degrees Fahrenheit. Lightly grease a 9x13 baking dish with olive oil. Lay it out on a baking pan

- Add 2 tablespoons olive oil to a large skillet placed over medium heat. When it begins to shimmer, add the garlic and cook until fragrant, about 1 minute. Stir in the spinach until it has wilted and most of the moisture has disappeared. Turn off the heat and remove from the pan.

- Arrange the bread cubes in a single layer on the pan's bottom. 13 of the cheeses, roasted red pepper, spinach, prosciutto, and scallions should be layered on top. Repeat the layering technique with more bread until all of the ingredients are used up.

- In a large mixing bowl, combine the eggs, milk, italian seasoning, salt, and pepper. It should be poured over the piled bread in the baking dish.

- Bake for 60 to 70 minutes, or until a knife inserted into the center comes out clean and the strata is puffed up and somewhat brown on top.

NOTES:

- For this recipe I use about ¾ of a large round loaf of bread.

- Use 2% instead of whole milk if that's what you have on hand

- To make this vegetarian, leave out the prosciutto.

- If you don't like chevre, substitute mozzarella.

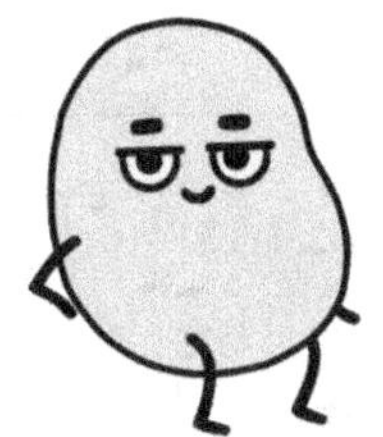

Leftover Mashed Potato Pancakes

 **PREP TIME:** 10 mins	 **COOK TIME:** 5 mins	 **SERVINGS:** 8 Servings	 **COURSE:** Appetizer, Breakfast or Side

Nutritional Value:	Calories: 146.5kcal	Fat: 2.9g	Carb: 25.3g	Protein: 5g

INGREDIENTS:

- Extra Virgin Olive Oil for pan frying
- 3 cups chilled mashed potatoes, already cooked and stored in the fridge
- ½ cup feta cheese, crumbled, more for garnish
- cup all-purpose flour
- 3 scallions, both white and green parts, chopped, plus more for garnish
- ¼ cup chopped fresh parsley
- 1 egg
- ⅓ to ½ cup plain breadcrumbs

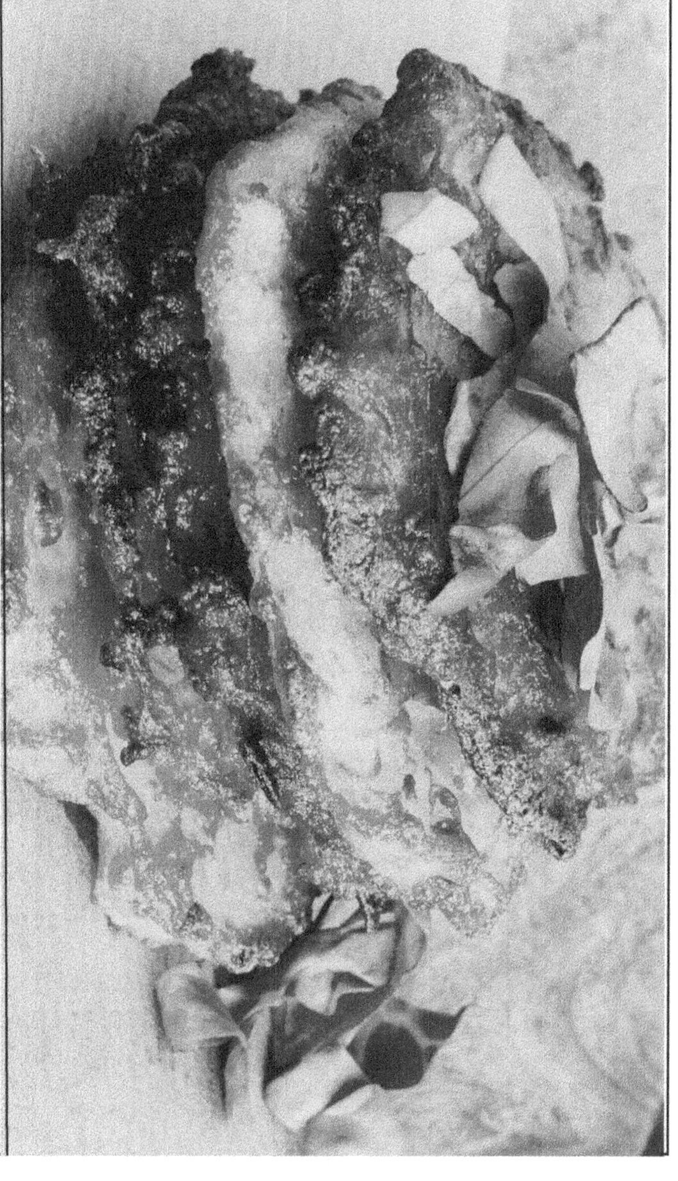

DIRECTIONS:

- To make the mashed potato mixture, combine the mashed potatoes, feta, all-purpose flour, scallions, and parsley in a large mixing basin. Break the egg and place it in the mixing bowl. Mix everything together with a wooden spoon until everything is properly combined.

- Spread the breadcrumbs on a plate and place it next to the bowl containing the mashed potato mixture.

- Make the patties as follows: Scoop a part of the mashed potato mixture to fill a measuring cup (14 cup or 13 cup, depending on the size of the patties you want). Form a ball with your hands, then lightly flatten into a 12-inch thick patty. Dredge the patty in breadcrumbs on both sides and place it flat on a baking sheet. Continue until the mashed potato mixture is done.

- To fry the mashed potato patties, prepare a large nonstick skillet or pan over medium-high heat. Fill the pan with olive oil until it is about 12 inches deep. When the oil shimmers, put the patties in a single layer in the pan (do this in batches if necessary). Cook for 2 to 3 minutes on one side, or until the bottom is crispy and golden brown, then flip and cook for another 2 to 3 minutes, watching for crisp and color on the second side.

- Remove the cooked mashed potato patties from the skillet with a spatula and place them on a plate lined with a paper towel to drain any leftover oil.

- Place the mashed potato patties on a serving platter and top with feta cheese and scallions. Enjoy!

NOTES:

- You may use any leftover mashed potatoes for this, such as our roasted garlic mashed potatoes, but you can also use our savory mashed sweet potatoes.

- My preferred cheese is feta, but feel free to substitute your favorite in this recipe.

- Serve leftover mashed potato pancakes with roast chicken for breakfast instead of hashbrowns.

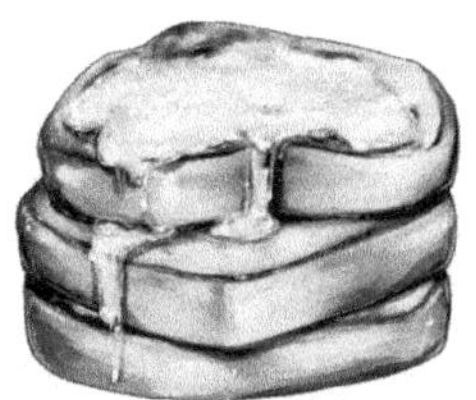

Challah French Toast with Orange Honey Syrup

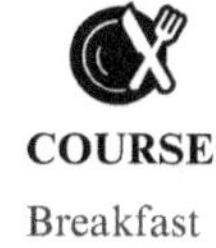

PREP TIME:	COOK TIME:	SERVINGS:	COURSE:
20 mins	10 mins	5 Servings	Breakfast

Nutritional Value:	Calories: 558.6kcal	Fat: 13g	Carb: 92.6g	Protein: 19g

INGREDIENTS:

For The Orange Honey Syrup:

- ½ cup honey
- ¼ cup orange juice
- 2 oranges, zested and supremed

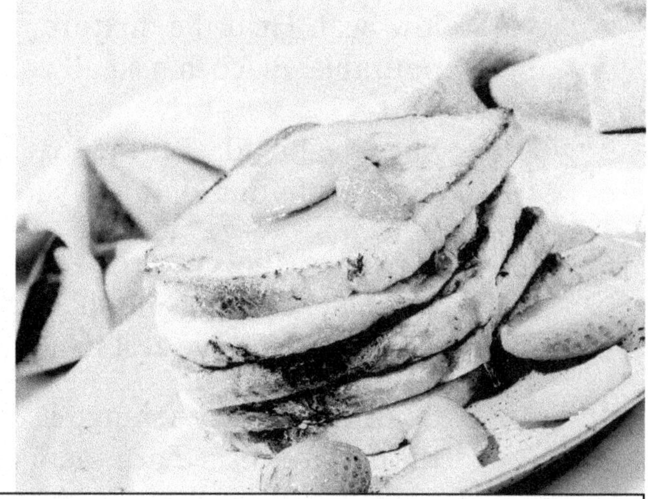

For The French Toast:

- 1 loaf challah bread, about 8 to 10 thick slices
- 6 eggs
- 1 cup whole milk
- 1 ¾ teaspoon ground cinnamon
- 1 teaspoon almond extract
- ¼ teaspoon kosher salt
- 4 teaspoons granulated sugar
- 1 cup blueberries
- 4 tablespoons creme fraiche, optional

DIRECTIONS:

- Supreme the oranges by zesting each orange and reserving the zest. Remove the top and bottom of an orange to create a flat surface on which to work and reveal the orange's flesh. Begin at the top and work your way down, slicing between the orange flesh and the white pith. Do this all the way around the orange until no peel or pith remains.

- Holding the orange over a small bowl to catch any fluids, carefully remove each segment from the membrane and place on a small dish. Rep with the other orange. After segmenting each orange, squeeze the membranes to release any juices into the bowl.

- Make the syrup as follows: 12 cup honey and 14 cup orange juice from when you supremed the oranges in a small pot set over medium low heat. Heat the mixture, stirring occasionally, until it is mixed and pourable. Place in a small container.

- Slice the bread: Cut the loaf into 12 inch thick wedges. Depending on the size of your loaf, you should finish up with 8 to 10 slices.

- To make the custard, follow these steps: Using a fork or whisk, combine the eggs, milk, ground cinnamon, almond extract, salt, sugar, and orange zest in a pie plate or wide shallow dish.

- Soak the bread: Arrange as many slices as will fit in a single layer in the custard dish. Turn them over to cover both sides.

- Heat the skillet: In a skillet over medium heat, melt 2 tablespoons butter or ghee. When it begins to sizzle, add the moistened bread in a single layer. Cook until golden brown on one side, then flip and cook until golden brown on the other.

- Place two slices of french toast on a dish to serve. 1 tablespoon cream fraiche, berries, and orange slices on top. Serve with the orange honey syrup drizzled on top. (If you have another orange on hand and are feeling fancy, zest some over the top of the toast before serving.)

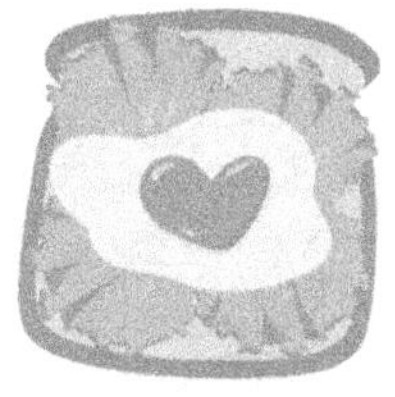

Egg Toast with Vegetables (Healthy Breakfast Recipe)

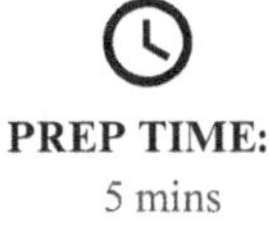

PREP TIME:
5 mins

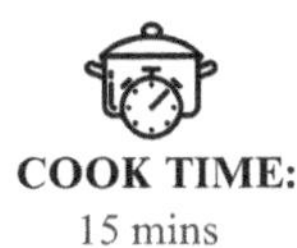

COOK TIME:
15 mins

SERVINGS:
4 Servings

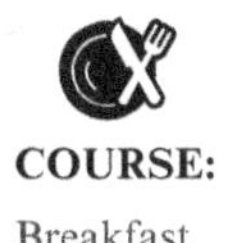

COURSE:
Breakfast

Nutritional Value:	Calories: 175.2kcal	Fat: 6.8g	Carb: 17.7g	Protein: 11.3g

INGREDIENTS:

- 4 to 5 large eggs
- Kosher salt
- ½ teaspoon sweet paprika
- ½ teaspoon red pepper flakes or 1 teaspoon Aleppo-style pepper
- 1 bell pepper, chopped
- ½ cup cherry tomatoes, halved or chopped
- 2 green onions, trimmed and chopped
- ¼ cup crumbled feta cheese
- 3 tablespoons chopped fresh parsley
- Extra virgin olive oil
- 4 slices of sandwich bread, thick cut

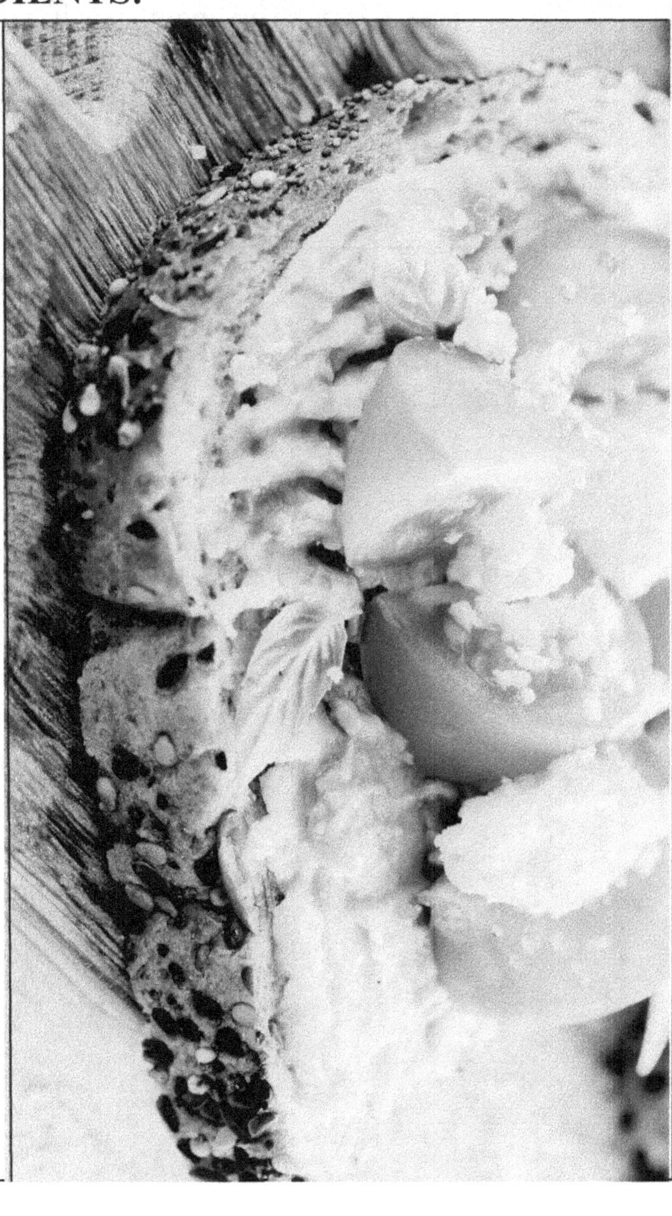

DIRECTIONS:

- Preheat the oven to 375°F and arrange a rack in the center.

- The eggs should be beaten and seasoned. Whisk the eggs in a medium mixing basin with kosher salt, paprika, red pepper flakes, or Aleppo-style pepper.

- Add the vegetables, and so forth. Add the vegetables, feta, and parsley, as well as a sprinkle of good extra virgin olive oil.

- Make the bread. Arrange the bread on a sheet pan brushed with olive oil.

- Top each slice of bread with a spoonful of the egg mixture.

- Bake. Place the sheet pan in the oven on the center rack. Bake for 15 minutes, or until the egg mixture is completely cooked and the vegetables have softened somewhat.

NOTES:

- Variations include finely chopped red onions instead of green onions, firm chopped Roma tomatoes in place of the cherry tomatoes, and different flavors such as smoky paprika or homemade Italian seasoning.

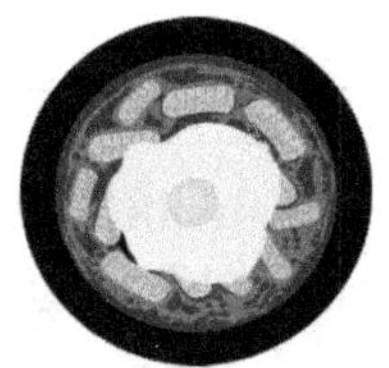

Eggs Fra Diavolo

	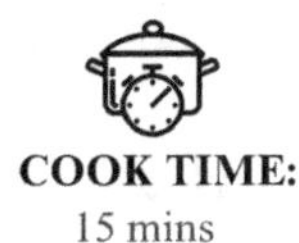		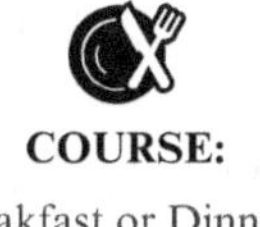
PREP TIME:	**COOK TIME:**	**SERVINGS:**	**COURSE:**
5 mins	15 mins	6	Breakfast or Dinner

Nutritional Value:	Calories: 101.2kcal	Fat: 5.5g	Carb: 5.7g	Protein: 7.4g

INGREDIENTS:

- Extra virgin olive oil
- 6 hardboiled eggs, peeled
- For The Spicy Tomato Sauce
- 1 medium onion, yellow or red, chopped
- 5 garlic cloves, minced
- 1 hot pepper such as jalapeño, chopped
- Kosher salt
- 1 5 ounce can diced fire-roasted tomatoes
- ¼ cup tomato paste
- 2 teaspoons dried oregano
- 1 to 2 teaspoon dried red pepper flakes or Aleppo pepper, more or less to your liking (if you like
- the sauce hot, you can add more)
- ½ cup basil or parsley, chopped

DIRECTIONS:

- Heat 2 tablespoons extra virgin olive oil in a 10-inch skillet or pan over medium-high heat until shimmering. Cook until the egg whites begin to crisp up and turn golden brown (put a splatter guard over your pan to protect the oil from splashing). Remove the eggs from the pan and place them on a plate or bowl for the time being.

- Add the onions, garlic, and jalapeno to the same pan. Cook for 3–5 minutes, tossing occasionally, until aromatic. Season with kosher salt to taste.

- Pour in the diced tomatoes, tomato paste, and 14 cup of water. Season with another generous pinch of kosher salt. If using, add the oregano and red pepper flakes. Bring the mixture to a boil, then reduce to a medium-low heat and let the tomatoes simmer for about 10 minutes.

- Cook for another 3 minutes, or until the eggs are warm, in the boiling tomato sauce.

- Remove from the fire and top with parsley and a generous drizzle of extra virgin olive oil. Serve with warm flatbread or crusty toast.

NOTES:

- Skip the boiled eggs if you want to make this recipe the traditional manner. Make the spicy tomato sauce first, then break 6 raw eggs and nestle them in it. Allow the sauce to continue to simmer until the egg whites have set and the yolks are creamy and slightly runny. This is similar to making shakshuka.

- The sauce is a twist on this fra diavolo recipe: I eliminated the white wine in today's recipe and substituted fresh chilies.

- Leftovers: Refrigerate leftovers in a firmly sealed glass jar for up to 3 days. Warm them up over medium heat, adding a little water if the sauce becomes too dry.

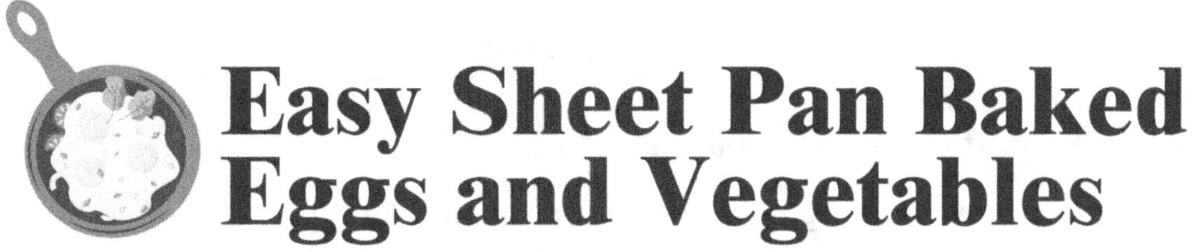

Easy Sheet Pan Baked Eggs and Vegetables

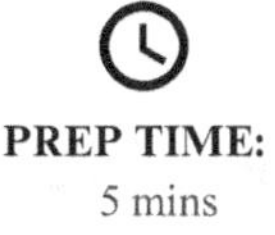

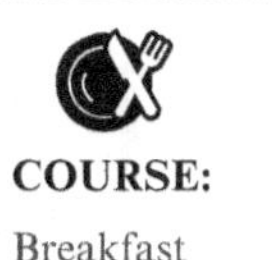

PREP TIME:	COOK TIME:	SERVINGS:	COURSE:
5 mins	15 mins	6 Servings	Breakfast

Nutritional Value:	Calories: 142.7kcal	Fat: 10.3g	Carb: 6g	Protein: 7.2g

INGREDIENTS:

- 1 green bell pepper, cored and thinly sliced
- 1 orange bell pepper, cored and thinly sliced
- 1 red bell pepper, cored and thinly sliced
- 1 medium red onion, halved then thinly sliced
- Kosher salt and black pepper
- Spices of your choice, I used 2 teaspoon za'atar blend, 1 teaspoon ground cumin and 1 teaspoon
- Aleppo chili pepper
- Extra virgin olive oil, I used Early Harvest Greek extra virgin olive oil
- 6 large eggs
- Chopped fresh parsley, a large handful
- 1 Roma tomato, diced
- Crumbled feta, a small bit to your liking (optional)

DIRECTIONS:

- Preheat the oven to 400 degrees Fahrenheit.

- In a large mixing bowl, combine sliced bell peppers of all hues. Add the red onions. 1 teaspoon za'atar, 1 teaspoon cumin, and 1 teaspoon Aleppo chili pepper (save the remaining za'atar for later). Drizzle with extra virgin olive oil to finish. To coat, toss with a fork

- Place the pepper and onion mixture on a large sheet pan. Spread in a single layer. Bake for 10 to 15 minutes in a preheated oven.

- Remove the pan from the oven for a few minutes. Make 6 "holes" or openings in the roasted vegetables. Carefully crack each egg into a hole, leaving the yoke intact (it helps to crack the egg in a tiny dish to slip into each hole carefully)

- Return the baking pan to the oven and bake until the egg whites have settled. Watch the yokes for 5 to 8 minutes to watch them transform to the doness you prefer.

- Take the pan out of the oven. Season the eggs to taste. Sprinkle with the remaining 1 teaspoon za'atar. Sprinkle with parsley, sliced tomatoes, and feta. Serve right away!

NOTES:

- Variations: You can truly customize this baked egg dish. Adapt the vegetables to what you have on hand. Adjust the roasting time as needed. Summer squash, zucchini, broccoli, cauliflower, and even root veggies might work.

- You can also experiment with different spice combinations. If you want smoky flavors, try some smoked paprika with salt and pepper. For a Moroccan touch, try harissa spice blend and a dash of turmeric. For an Italian touch, add dried oregano or basil. Before adding the eggs, add some cooked meat (such as chorizo, Italian sausage, or leftover rotisserie chicken) to the sheet pan with the roasted vegetables.

- Preparation Hints: This is a simple enough recipe to cook on the day you intend to serve it. It will look best then, but if you want to try to work ahead, prep the peppers and onions ahead of time and store them in the fridge overnight.

You may also roast the vegetables the night before. Refrigerate them in a container with a tight-fitting lid. When ready, spread on a sheet pan and continue with the recipe from step 5. It's not ideal because you'll have to clean the sheet pan twice.

Leftovers can be stored in the fridge for up to three days.To store, split leftovers into glass containers with tight covers and chill for whatever many meals you intend to make. At room temperature or warmed through, this dish is delicious. Warm in a skillet over medium heat for a few minutes.

Can sheet pan eggs be frozen? No, not in this recipe. When frozen, sunny side up eggs lose texture and flavor

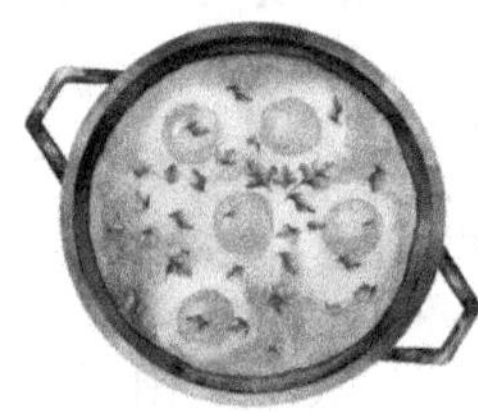# Easy Shakshuka Recipe

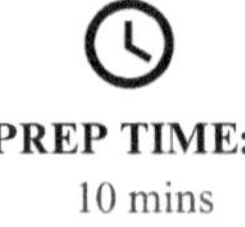 **PREP TIME:** 10 mins	 **COOK TIME:** 30 mins	 **SERVINGS:** 6	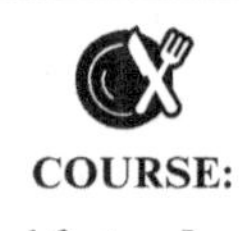 **COURSE:** Breakfast or Lunch

Nutritional Value:	Calories: 111kcal	Fat: 4.7g	Carb: 10.9g	Protein: 7.7g

INGREDIENTS:

- Extra virgin olive oil
- 1 large yellow onion chopped
- 2 green peppers chopped
- 2 garlic cloves, chopped
- 1 teaspoon ground coriander
- 1 teaspoon sweet paprika
- ½ teaspoon ground cumin
- Pinch red pepper flakes optional
- Salt and pepper
- 6 medium tomatoes, chopped (about 6 cups chopped tomatoes)
- ½ cup tomato sauce
- 6 large eggs
- ¼ cup chopped fresh parsley leaves
- ¼ cup chopped fresh mint leaves

DIRECTIONS:

- In a large cast iron skillet, heat 3 tablespoons olive oil. Add the onions, green peppers, garlic, spices, and a bit of salt and pepper to taste. Cook, stirring periodically, for 5 minutes, or until the veggies have softened.

- Combine the tomatoes and tomato sauce in a mixing bowl. Allow to simmer for about 15 minutes, covered. Uncover and continue to simmer for a few minutes longer to allow the mixture to decrease and thicken. Season with salt and pepper to taste.

- Make 6 indentations, or "wells," in the tomato mixture using a wooden spoon (make sure the indentations are evenly spaced). Crack an egg into each indentation gently.

- Reduce the heat to low, cover the skillet, and simmer until the egg whites are firm.

- Remove the cover and stir in the fresh parsley and mint. If desired, season with additional black pepper or crushed red pepper. Serve with warm pita, challah, or your favorite crusty bread.

NOTES:

- Make-Ahead Tip: You may make the shakshuka tomato sauce the night before. Allow it cool completely before storing in a glass container with a tight lid in the refrigerator. When you're ready, heating up the sauce in a skillet, add the eggs, and continue with the recipe from step #3.

- Leftovers will stay in the fridge for 1 to 2 days if stored carefully in tight-lid glass containers. Warm the shakshuka sauce over medium heat, adding a little more liquid if necessary.

- Cook around 12 ground beef or ground lamb in extra virgin olive oil if you want to add meat. Season with salt and pepper to taste. Remove the meat from the skillet, wipe it clean, and repeat steps #1 and #2 to prepare the shakshuka sauce, but this time add the cooked ground meat to the skillet to simmer with the tomatoes for about 15 minutes before adding the eggs.

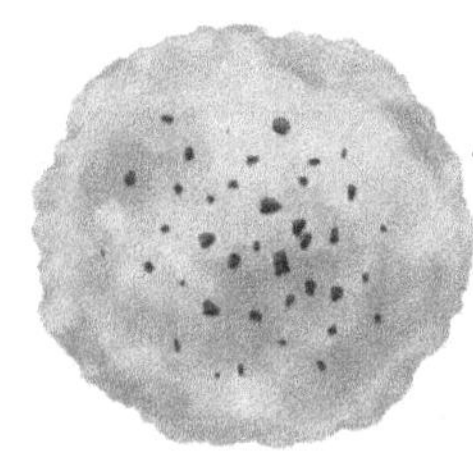

Easy Potato Omelet Recipe

 **PREP TIME:** 5 mins	 **COOK TIME:** 15 mins	 **SERVINGS:** 6	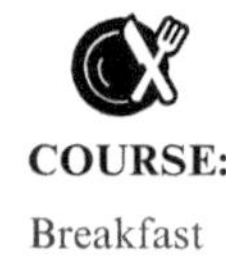 **COURSE:** Breakfast

Nutritional Value:	Calories: 176.2kcal	Fat: 9.1g	Carb: 16.4g	Protein: 7.7g

INGREDIENTS:

- Extra virgin olive oil
- 3 gold potatoes, about 12 ounces, peeled and cut into ½-inch cubes
- 1 to 2 green onions, both whites and greens, sliced into rounds
- 1 to 2 garlic cloves, minced
- Kosher salt
- 1 teaspoon coriander
- 1 teaspoon Aleppo pepper
- ½ teaspoon sweet paprika
- ¼ teaspoon turmeric
- 6 large eggs
- ½ cup chopped fresh dill
- ½ cup chopped fresh parsley

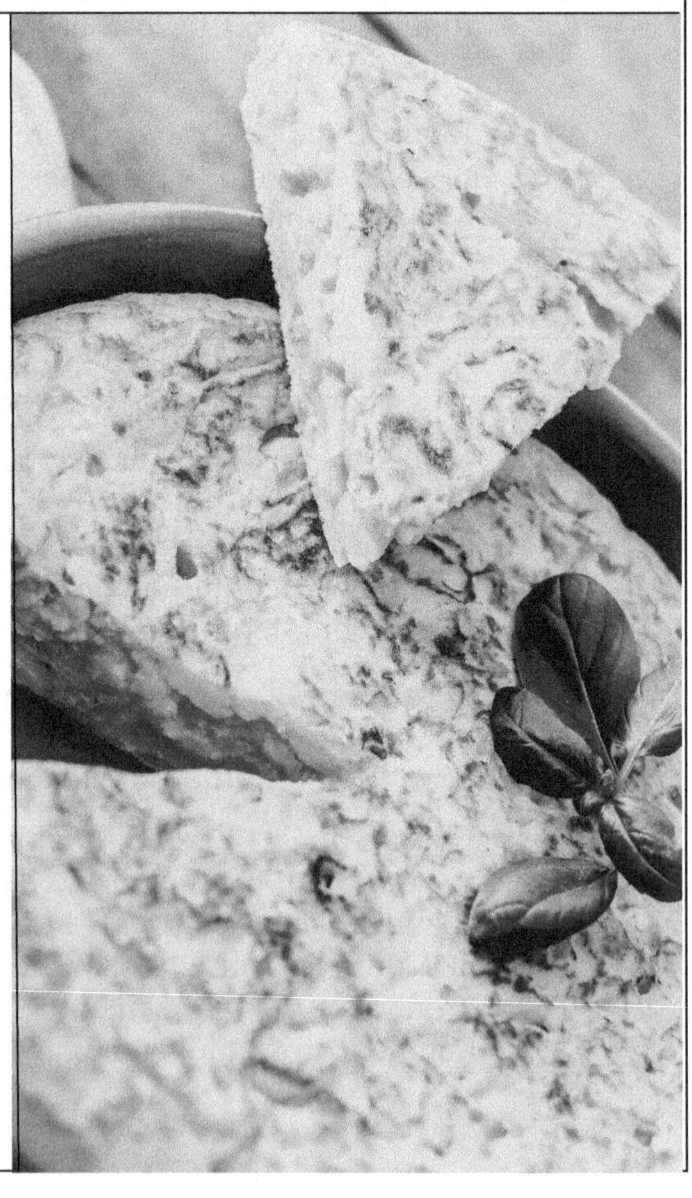

DIRECTIONS:

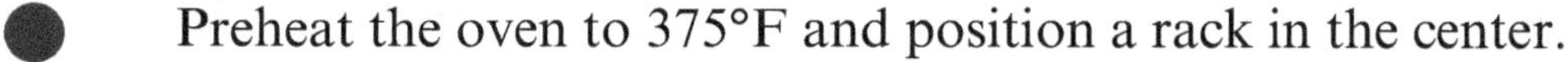

- Preheat the oven to 375°F and position a rack in the center.

- Heat roughly 2 tablespoons extra virgin olive oil in a 10-inch cast iron or oven-safe pan over mediumhigh heat until shimmering but not smoking.

- Combine the diced potatoes, green onions, and garlic in a mixing bowl. Kosher salt, coriander, Aleppo pepper, paprika, and turmeric to taste. Cook, stirring frequently, for 5 to 10 minutes, or until the potatoes are soft and cooked through (manage the heat to prevent the garlic from burning).

- Pour the egg mixture over the potatoes in the skillet and cook until the edges and bottom have settled somewhat (approximately 3 to 4 minutes).

- Place the skillet in the preheated oven. Bake for 8 to 10 minutes, or until the eggs are fully cooked through and the top is no longer runny.

NOTES:

- Substitutions: You can use russet or sweet potatoes if you do not have gold potatoes.

- Salt the eggs before cooking them

- Add ¼ teaspoon baking powder to the egg mixture for fluffy eggs

- The potato omelet can be served hot or cold

- Vegetables or a salad, such as lemon-garlic sautéed asparagus, grilled zucchini salad, 3 bean salad, or fennel orange salad, go well with it.

- Leftovers and storage: Refrigerate this cooked omelet with potatoes in an airtight container for 3 to 4 days. To reheat, lay the omelet on a baking sheet and place in the center rack of a 350°F oven until warmed through (about 5 minutes).

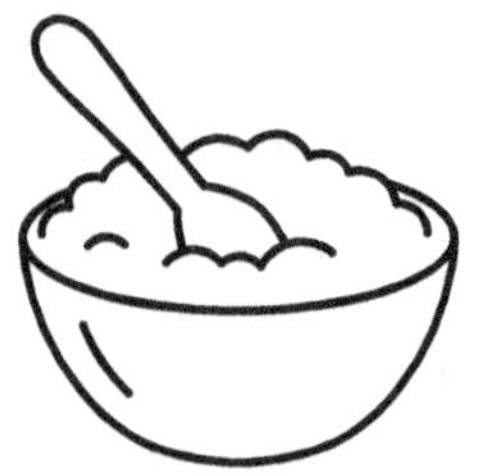

Easy Savory Oatmeal Bowls Recipe

 **PREP TIME:** 5 mins	 **COOK TIME:** 15 mins	 **SERVINGS:** 6 Bowls	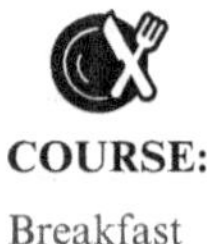 **COURSE:** Breakfast

Nutritional Value:	Calories: 348.2kcal	Fat: 14.1g	Carb: 42.6g	Protein: 13.7g

INGREDIENTS:

- 1 medium yellow onion, chopped
- 1 sweet potato, about 1 pound, peeled and chopped into ½-inch cubes
- Kosher salt and black pepper
- 1 cup quick-cooking steel-cut oats
- 4 eggs
- 1 avocado, optional, cut into small cubes
- 1 cup cherry tomatoes, halved
- ½ cup chopped fresh parsley
- Feta cheese, crumbled
- Za'atar
- 2 tablespoons extra virgin olive oil

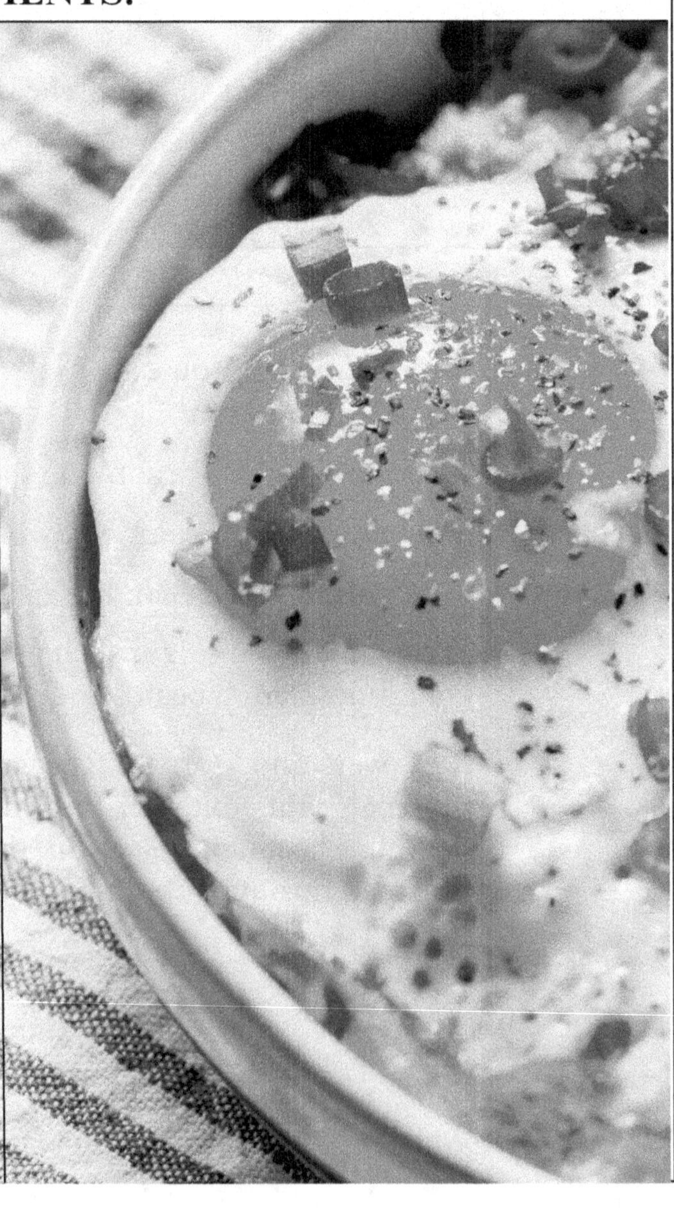

DIRECTIONS:

- Heat about 2 tablespoons extra virgin olive oil in a large nonstick skillet. Combine the sweet potatoes and onions in a mixing bowl. Season with kosher salt and freshly ground black pepper to taste. Cook for 5 minutes, tossing occasionally, over medium-high heat. Cook for another 5 to 7 minutes, or until the potatoes are soft.

- Cook your quick-cooking steel cut oatmeal according to package directions (mine required 2 cups of boiling water and around 5 minutes to cook), stirring periodically. Season with kosher salt to taste.

- Cook the eggs to your preference. I like to fry my eggs sunny side up in extra virgin olive oil.

- Put together the savory oats bowls. In the bowl, place some cooked oats. Mix in the sweet potatoes, avocado cubes, and cooked egg. Finish with a handful of tomatoes, parsley, feta, and a sprinkling of za'atar or your favorite seasoning. Serve right away.

NOTES:

Make-ahead tips:

- Cook the sweet potatoes ahead of time (1 or 2 nights ahead) and store them in a tightly sealed jar in the refrigerator. Better still, if you have cooked vegetables on hand, use them instead of starting from scratch (I frequently use leftover roasted sweet potatoes in these bowls).

- Cook the oatmeal the night before and refrigerate it. Because oatmeal hardens in the fridge, you'll need to add extra liquid when reheating it (see instructions below).

- When you're ready to eat, just fry your egg, crumble your feta, and construct your savory oatmeal bowl.

Leftovers and storage

- Refrigerate all leftovers in separate airtight containers. Cooked oatmeal with sweet potatoes can be stored for 3 to 5 days.

- In a saucepan over medium heat, reheat sweet potatoes.

- To reheat oats, place them in a small saucepan with a splash of water to help loosen them up. Warm over low to medium-low heat, adding more liquid as needed, until the oats regain their creamy consistency. If you like overnight oats, they will also work! Simply reheat them in the manner stated above.

Çılbır: Turkish Poached Eggs

PREP TIME:
10 mins

COOK TIME:
10 mins

SERVINGS:
2 Servings

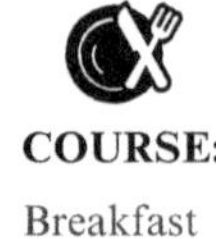

COURSE:
Breakfast

Nutritional Value:	Calories: 343.8kcal	Fat: 5.7g	Carb: 6.3g	Protein: 17.2g

INGREDIENTS:

- 1 cup plain Greek yogurt (made with whole milk, at room temperature)
- 1 to 2 garlic cloves (finely minced)
- 2 eggs
- 3 tablespoons extra virgin olive oil
- 1 to 2 tablespoons vinegar (optional)
- 2 teaspoons Aleppo pepper (or red pepper flakes)

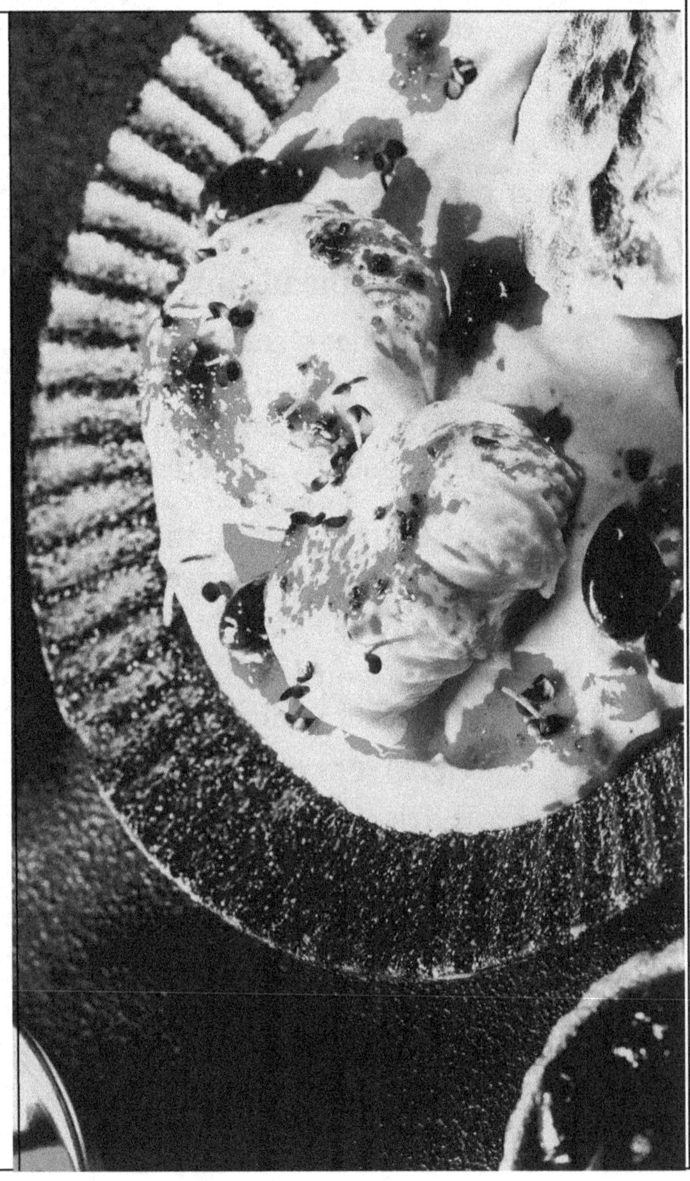

DIRECTIONS:

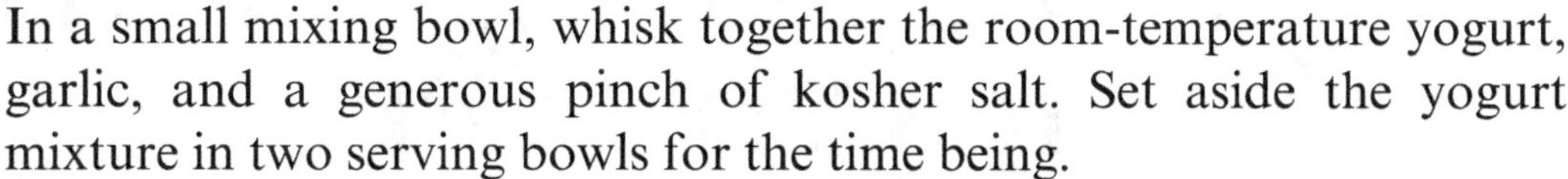

In a small mixing bowl, whisk together the room-temperature yogurt, garlic, and a generous pinch of kosher salt. Set aside the yogurt mixture in two serving bowls for the time being.

Bring a small saucepan of water to a boil. Add the vinegar and mix well.

Meanwhile, place an egg in a fine mesh sieve set over a small bowl. Gently swirl the eggs in the sieve to drain the liquidy part of the egg whites (this results in a more aesthetically pleasing poached egg). Place the egg in a ramekin.

When the water is ready, swirl it with a wooden spoon to produce a vortex. Add the egg to the center of the vortex and cook for 2 to 3 minutes. When the egg is done, move it to a dish lined with parchment paper using a slotted spoon.

Prepare and cook the second egg in the same manner as the first.

Make the olive oil sauce quickly while the second egg is frying. Warm the olive oil and Aleppo pepper in a small skillet over medium heat.

Transfer the poached eggs to the yogurt bowls right away (just place each egg on top of the yogurt mixture) and sprinkle with the hot oil.

Serve with your favorite rustic bread right away.

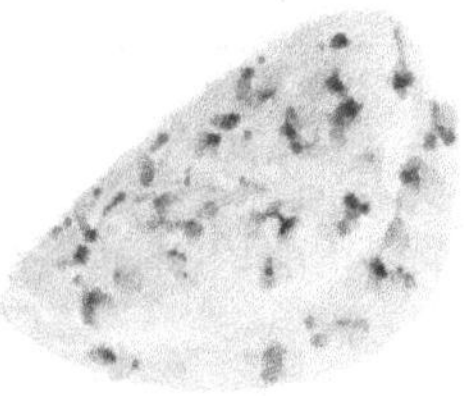

Za'atar Eggs Fried in Olive Oil

 **PREP TIME:** 1 min	 **COOK TIME:** 10 mins	 **SERVINGS:** 1 Egg	 **COURSE:** Breakfast

Nutritional Value:	Calories: 192.2kcal	Fat: 3.4g	Carb: 1.6g	Protein: 5.7g

INGREDIENTS:

- 1 large egg
- 1 to 2 tbsp extra virgin olive oil, more if you like
- ¼ teaspoon Kosher salt
- 2 tsp za'atar

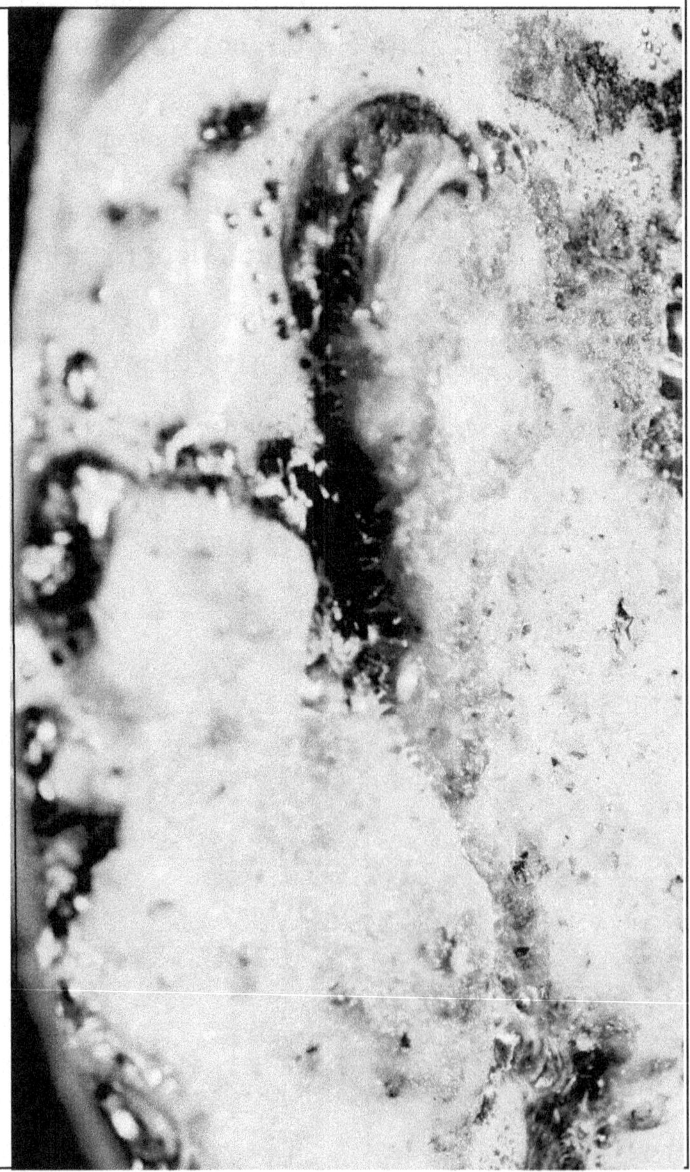

DIRECTIONS:

- In a ramekin or small dish, crack your egg.

- Warm a nonstick skillet over medium heat. Turn the heat to medium and add the olive oil. Tilt the pan to distribute the oil and watch for it to shimmy.

- Slide the eggs into the hot oil with care. Season with Kosher salt and za'atar to taste. Cook for 2 to 3 minutes over medium heat, spooning some olive oil on top, until the whites are done, the edges crisp up, and the yolk is cooked to your taste (if desired, cover the pan for a few seconds).

- Serve with warmed pita bread or your favorite crusty bread right away!

NOTES:

- I prefer my eggs to be swimming in nice EVOO, so I use extra. However, you can adjust the amount of olive oil to your desire.

- Add-ons: I like to add a few chopped cherry tomatoes and perhaps a little of feta. You can add them as soon as you finish seasoning your eggs in step 3.

- How long should you cook your egg? It will take approximately 2 to 2 12 minutes for a runny yolk and 3 minutes for a medium yolk. If you want to cook your eggs until the yolk solidifies, cover the skillet for a couple minutes and keep an eye on it until the yolk is cooked to your liking.

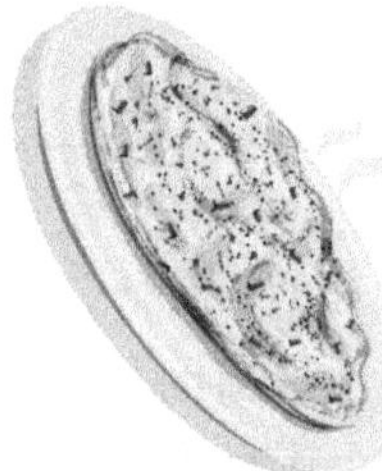

Menemen Recipe (Turkish Scrambled Eggs with Tomatoes)

 **PREP TIME:** 10 mins	 **COOK TIME:** 15 mins	 **SERVINGS:** 4 People	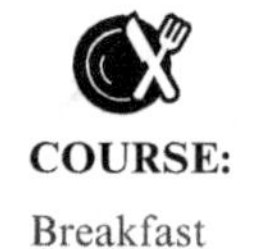 **COURSE:** Breakfast

Nutritional Value:	Calories: 164.7kcal	Fat: 11.5g	Carb: 9.3g	Protein: 7.2g

INGREDIENTS:

- 2 tablespoons extra virgin olive oil
- 1 medium yellow onion chopped
- 1 green bell pepper (Anaheim or Holland peppers will work as well), cored, seeded and chopped
- Kosher salt
- 2 vine-ripe tomatoes
- 3 tablespoons tomato paste
- Black pepper
- ½ teaspoon dried oregano
- 1 teaspoon Aleppo pepper, more for later
- 4 large eggs, beaten
- Crushed red pepper flakes, optional if you like spicy
- 1 French baguette for serving thickly sliced (optional)

DIRECTIONS:

Heat 2 tablespoons in a 10-inch pan over medium heat. Season the onions and peppers with kosher salt. Cook for 4 to 5 minutes, stirring frequently, until softened (but don't brown the onions).

Combine the tomatoes and tomato paste in a mixing bowl. Season with kosher salt, black pepper, oregano, and Aleppo pepper to taste. Cook, stirring periodically, for a few minutes over medium heat, until the tomatoes soften but retain their shape (5 to 7 minutes).

To one side of the pan, place the tomato and pepper mixture. Turn the heat down to medium-low. Cook for a few minutes, stirring gently as needed, until the eggs are just set. Incorporate the tomato mixture into the eggs.

Finish with a drizzle of EVOO and additional Aleppo pepper and crushed red pepper flakes, if desired. Serve with thick pieces of bread right away.

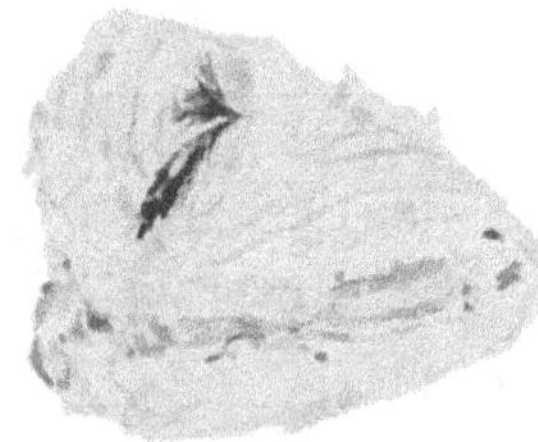

Kuku Sabzi: Persian Baked Omelet

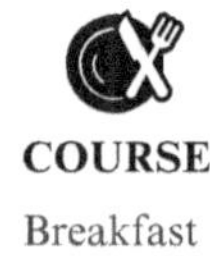

PREP TIME: 20 mins	**COOK TIME:** 20 mins	**SERVINGS:** 6	**COURSE:** Breakfast

Nutritional Value:	Calories: 184kcal	Fat: 16.7g	Carb: 3.1g	Protein: 7.1g

INGREDIENTS:

- 5 tbsp Private Reserve Greek extra virgin olive oil
- 2 cups flat-leaf parsley, leaves
- 2 cups cilantro, leaves and tender stems
- 1 cup roughly chopped fresh dill
- 6 scallions, trimmed and coarsely chopped
- 1 ½ tsp baking powder
- 1 tsp kosher salt
- ¾ tsp ground green cardamom
- ¾ tsp ground cinnamon
- ½ tsp ground cumin
- ¼ tsp ground black pepper
- 6 large eggs
- ½ cup walnuts, toasted and chopped (optional)
- ⅓ cup dried cranberries, coarsely chopped (optional)
- Cook Mode Prevent your screen from going dark

DIRECTIONS:

- Preheat the oven to 375°F and place an oven rack in the upper-middle position.

- Trace the bottom of an 8-inch square or 9-inch circular cake pan on kitchen parchment, then cut inside the lines to make a piece that fits in the pan.

- Coat the bottom and sides of the pan with 2 tablespoons extra virgin olive oil, flipping the parchment to coat on both sides (the oil should pool at the bottom and coat the sides generously).

- Combine the parsley, cilantro, dill, scallions, and the remaining 3 tablespoons extra virgin olive oil in a food processor. Process until finely ground (I prefer my herbs less fine, so I stopped the machine when I reached the desired texture). Set aside for the time being.

- Whisk together the baking powder, salt, cardamom, cinnamon, cumin, and pepper in a large mixing basin. Whisk in 2 eggs until incorporated, then add the remaining eggs and whisk until just combined. Fold in the herb-scallion mixture and, if using, the walnuts and cranberries. Smooth the top of the batter into the prepared pan.

- Bake at 375 degrees F for 20 to 25 minutes, or until the core of the egg is hard. (The egg mixture will rise first, but will fall once left aside to cool.)

- Allow the kuku to cool in the pan for 10 minutes, undisturbed. When ready, use a thin knife to loosen the kuku around the edges. Remove the parchment off the bottom of the kuku and invert onto another serving dish or cutting board so the top of the kuku is facing you. Serve warm or at room temperature, cut into wedges.

- Serve with a dollop of yogurt on the side. More ideas can be found in the section titled "what to serve with kuku sabzi.

NOTES:

- Milk Street: The New Home Cooking recipe used with permission from Milk Street.

- This recipe calls for our Private Reserve Greek extra virgin olive oil (made from sustainably produced and processed Koroneiki olives). SAVE! Consider our Greek Olive Oil Bundle!

LUNCH

RECIPES

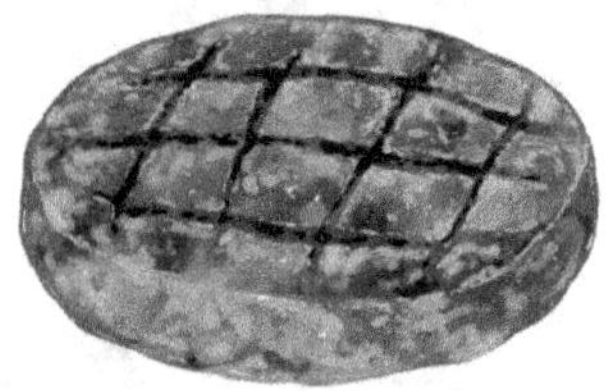

Tuna Patties Fried in Olive Oil (France)

 **PREP TIME:** 10 mins	 **COOK TIME:** 15 mins	 **SERVINGS:** 4	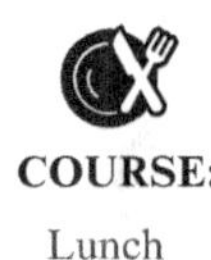 **COURSE:** Lunch

Nutritional Value:	Calories: 399kcal	Fat: 20g	Carb: 18g	Protein: 36g

INGREDIENTS:

- 2-7 ounces cans tuna
- 1/3 cup bread crumbs
- 2 shallots, chopped
- 1 tbsp parsley, chopped
- 3 tbsp chives, chopped
- 1 tbsp scallions, chopped
- 1/3 cup parmesan, grated
- 1/3 cup all purpose flour + 2 Tablespoons
- 1 tbsp sour cream
- 1 egg
- Salt and pepper, to taste
- 2 tbsp extra virgin olive oil

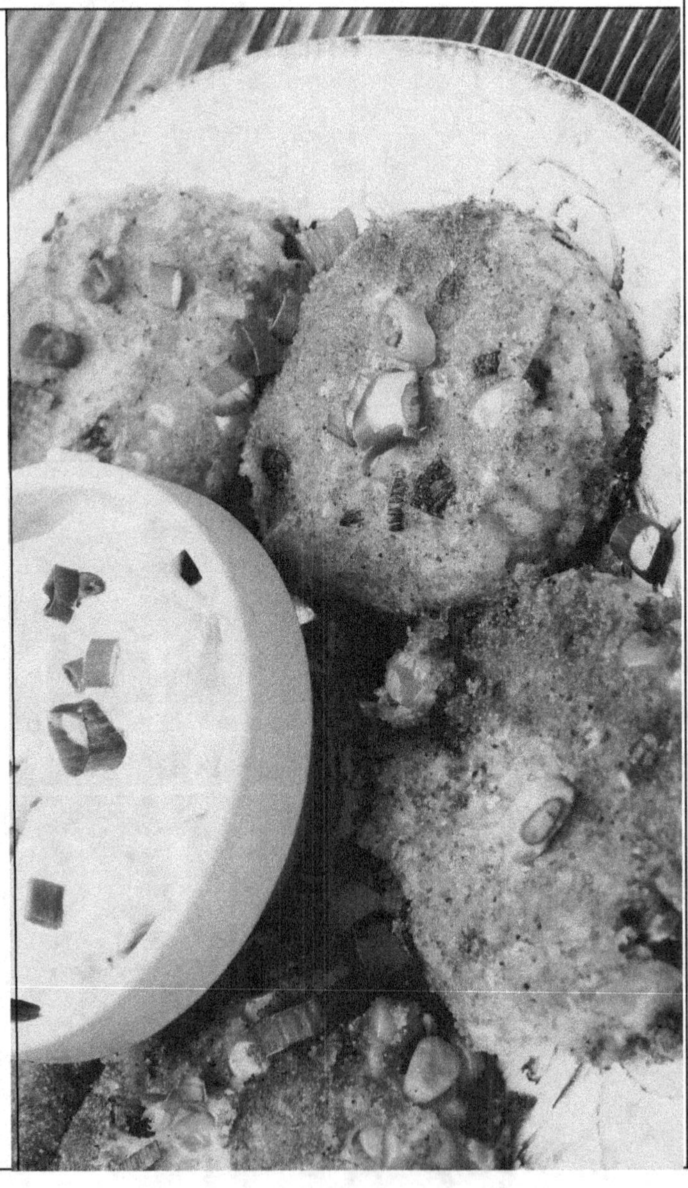

DIRECTIONS:

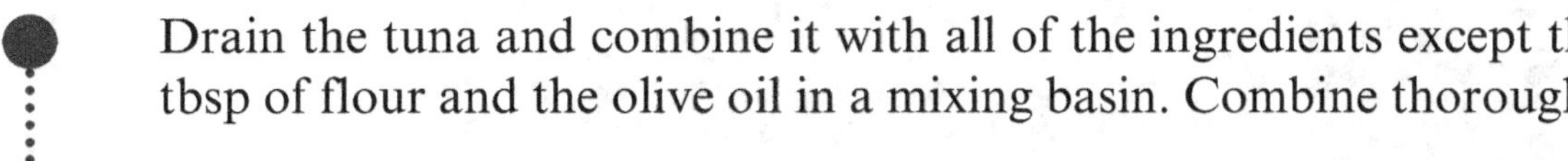

- Drain the tuna and combine it with all of the ingredients except the 2 tbsp of flour and the olive oil in a mixing basin. Combine thoroughly.

- On a small plate, place the 2 tablespoons of flour. Form medium patties, then roll them in the flour to coat lightly.

- Heat the olive oil in a frying pan over medium heat. Cook the patties for 7 minutes per side, or until lightly browned.

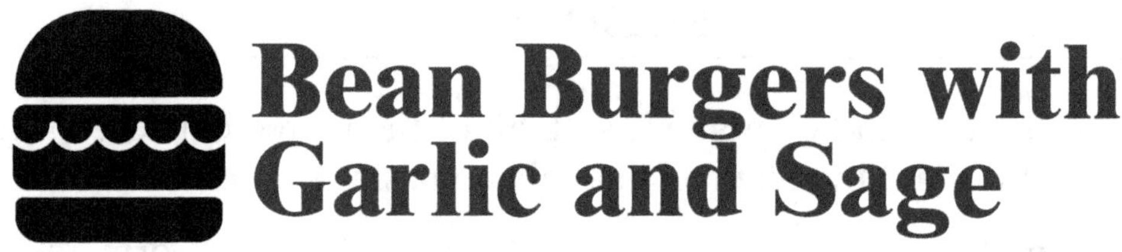

Bean Burgers with Garlic and Sage

PREP TIME: 10 mins	**COOK TIME:** 10 mins	**SERVINGS:** 2	**COURSE:** Lunch

Nutritional Value:	Calories: 305kcal	Fat: 25g	Carb: 14g	Protein: 7g

INGREDIENTS:

- 1-29 ounces can pink beans, rinsed and drained
- 1/2 onion minced
- 2 eggs
- 1 cup parsley, chopped
- 3/4 cup chickpea flour
- 1/2 tsp black pepper
- 1/2 tsp dried sage
- 1 tsp salt
- 1 tsp oregano, dried
- 2 cloves garlic, minced or pressed
- 1/2 cup Olive oil to fry

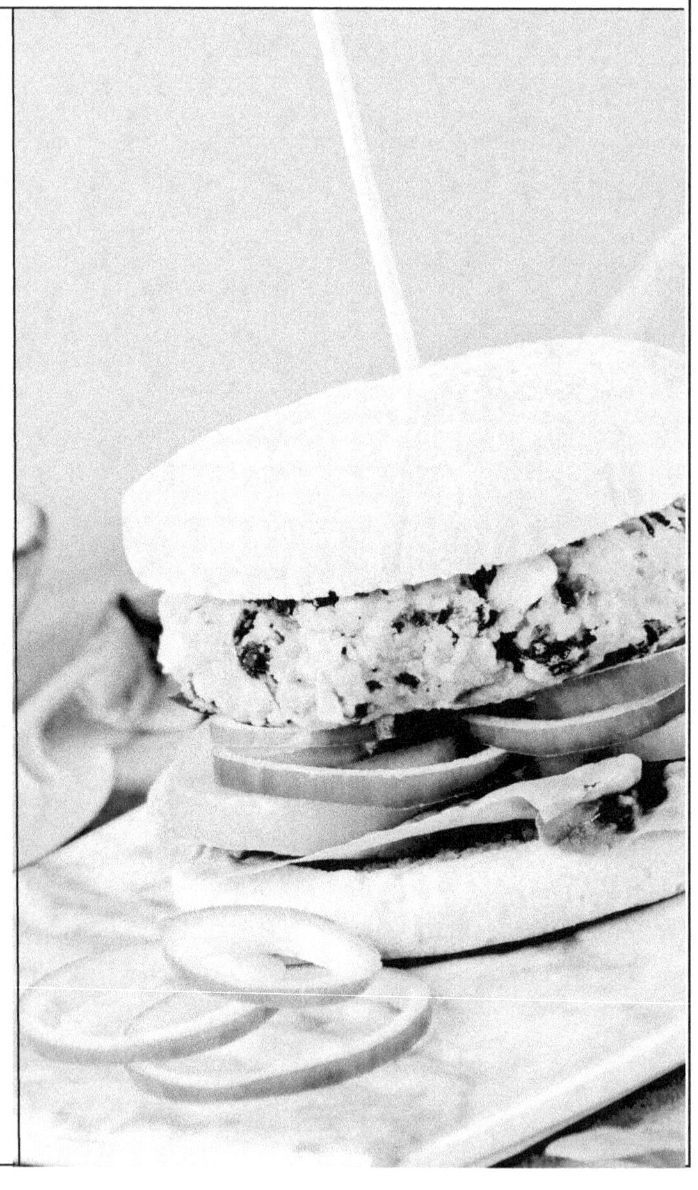

DIRECTIONS:

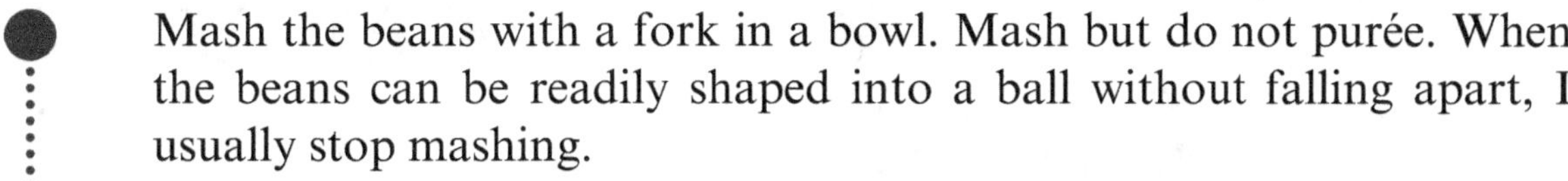

- Mash the beans with a fork in a bowl. Mash but do not purée. When the beans can be readily shaped into a ball without falling apart, I usually stop mashing.

- Combine all of the remaining ingredients (except the olive oil). Using a fork, thoroughly combine all ingredients.

- Heat the oil over medium heat. Make patties out of the bean mixture. Fry till golden brown on one side, then flip and repeat on the other. Dry with paper towels.

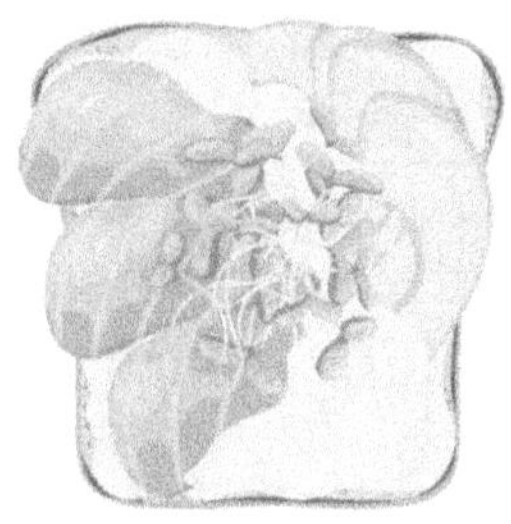

Avocado Toast with Caramelized Balsamic Onions

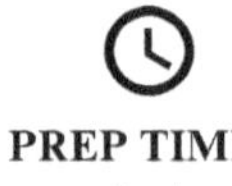 **PREP TIME:** 5 mins	 **COOK TIME:** 20 mins	 **SERVINGS:** 2	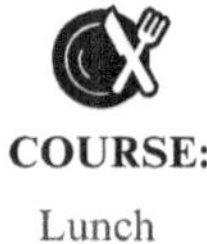 **COURSE:** Lunch

Nutritional Value:	Calories: 305kcal	Fat: 25g	Carb: 14g	Protein: 7g

INGREDIENTS:

- 2 tablespoons extra virgin olive oil
- 1 onion, sliced
- salt and pepper, to taste
- 1 tsp dried oregano
- 2 tbsp Balsamic vinegar
- 1 ripe avocado
- 2 slices toast

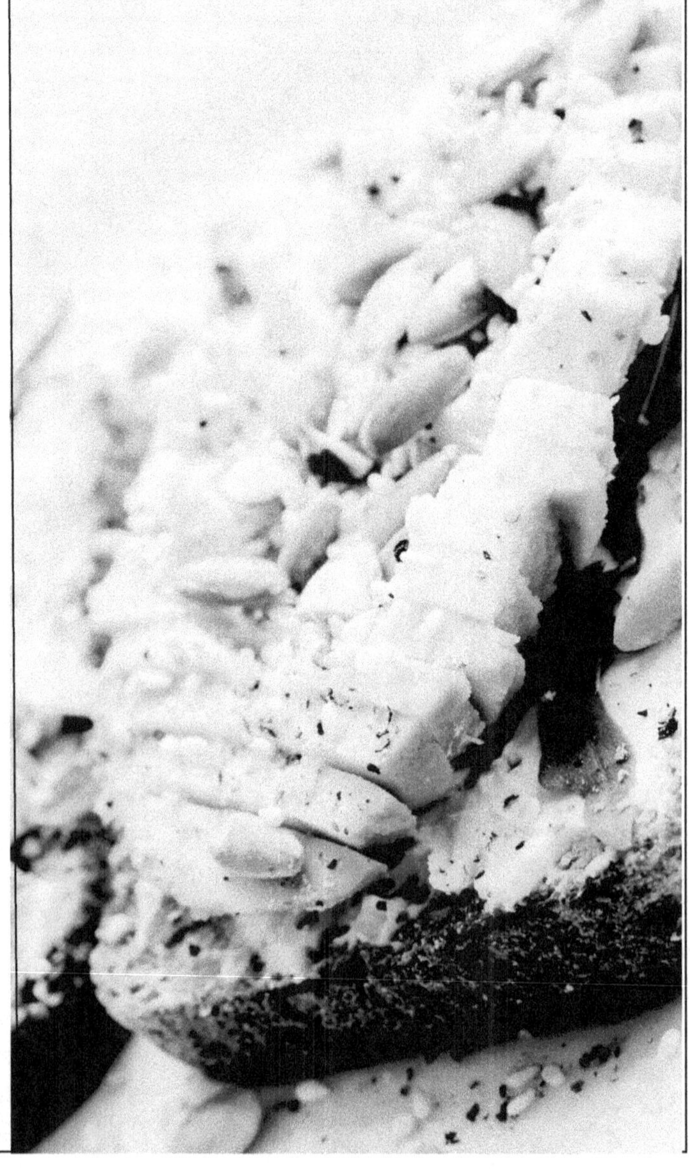

DIRECTIONS:

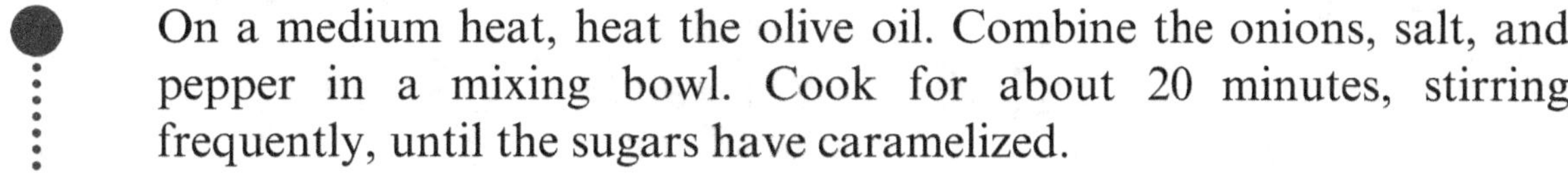

- On a medium heat, heat the olive oil. Combine the onions, salt, and pepper in a mixing bowl. Cook for about 20 minutes, stirring frequently, until the sugars have caramelized.

- Cook for 2 minutes after adding the balsamic vinegar to the onions. Take the pan off the heat.

- Mash the avocado, oregano, salt, and pepper in a mixing dish with a fork until smooth.

- Toast two slices of bread. Serve with the avocado mixture on top. Enjoy with caramelized onions on top!

Pasta Alla Puttanesca with Canned Tuna

PREP TIME: 5 mins	**COOK TIME:** 15 mins	**SERVINGS:** 2	**COURSE:** Lunch or Dinner

Nutritional Value:	Calories: 661kcal	Fat: 24g	Carb: 75g	Protein: 33g

INGREDIENTS:

- 6 oz dried pasta long varieties work best
- 1 small red onion thinly sliced
- 2 tbsp extra virgin olive oil
- 1 dried chili pepper minced (or more, according to your taste)
- 3 anchovy fillets in oil
- 1/8 cup white wine
- 8 oz cherry tomatoes cut in half
- 1 tbsp brined capers
- 1/4 cup black olives
- 5 oz canned tuna in oil drained
- 1/4 tsp oregano

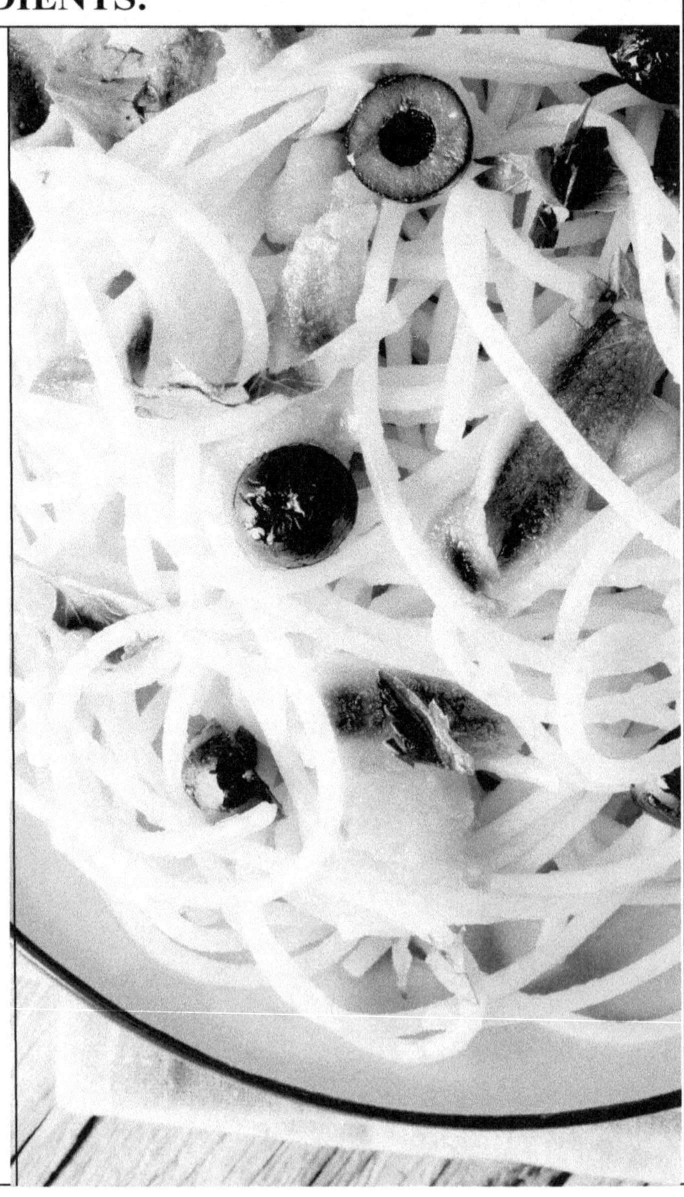

DIRECTIONS:

- A large pot of water should be brought to a boil. When it begins to boil, add salt and cook the pasta according to package guidelines.

- In the meantime, make the sauce. Combine the olive oil, chile pepper, and anchovy fillets in a large frying pan. Heat on medium-low for a few seconds, stirring constantly, until the anchovies are completely dissolved.

- Cook for 5 minutes, or until the onions begin to turn translucent, on medium heat

- Wait for the white wine to be absorbed after deglazing the pan.

- Combine the cherry tomatoes, capers, olives, and canned tuna in a mixing bowl. Cook for 8 to 10 minutes on medium-low heat. If the sauce becomes too dry, add a half-ladle of pasta water.

- When the pasta is al dente, drain it and add it to the pan with the sauce and oregano.

- Toss everything for 60 seconds, then remove from the heat and serve.

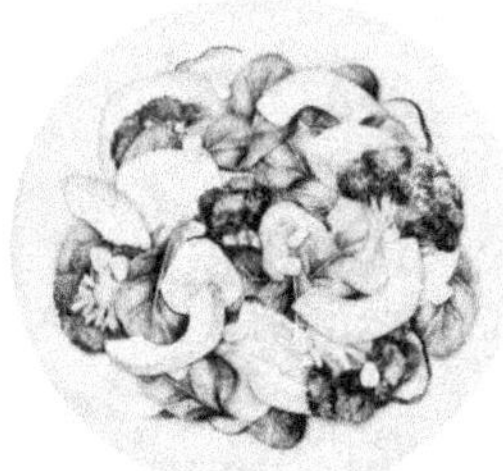

Avocado Salad with Cucumber and Radish

 **PREP TIME:** 15 mins

 **COOK TIME:** 0 mins

 **SERVINGS:** 4

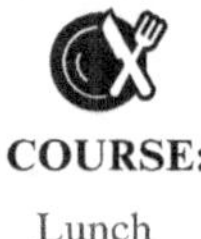 **COURSE:** Lunch

Nutritional Value:	Calories: 188kcal	Fat: 18g	Carb: 7g	Protein: 2g

INGREDIENTS:

- 2 medium radishes, chopped
- 1 large cucumber, cut into quarters lengthwise and then chopped
- 1/4 cup red onion, chopped
- 1 ripe avocado, cut into small chunks
- 1/4 cup chopped fresh parsley
- 1/2 lemon juice
- 1/2 tsp dried dill
- 3 tbsp extra virgin olive oil
- salt, to taste

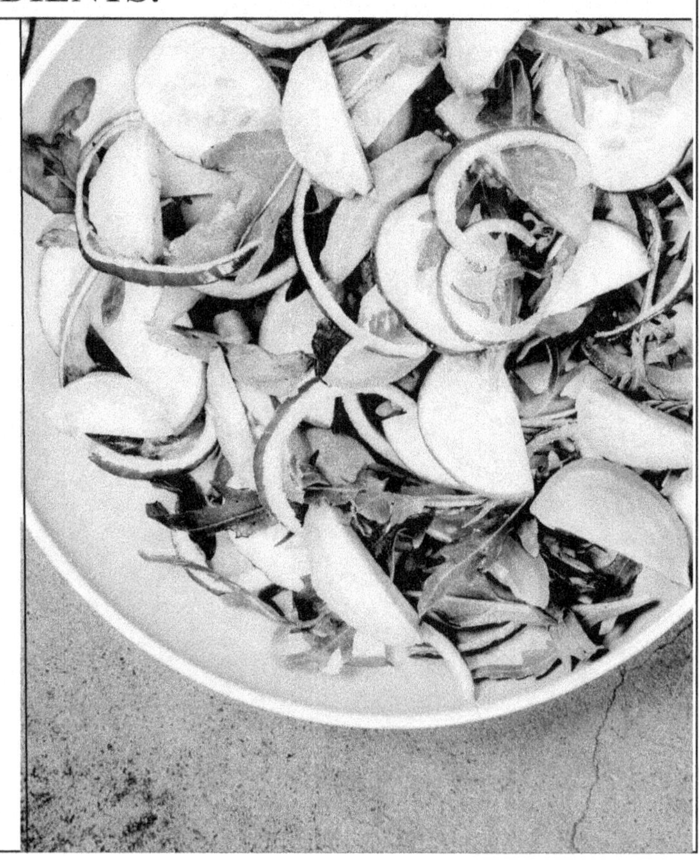

DIRECTIONS:

- In a large salad bowl, combine all of the ingredients. Toss thoroughly before serving.

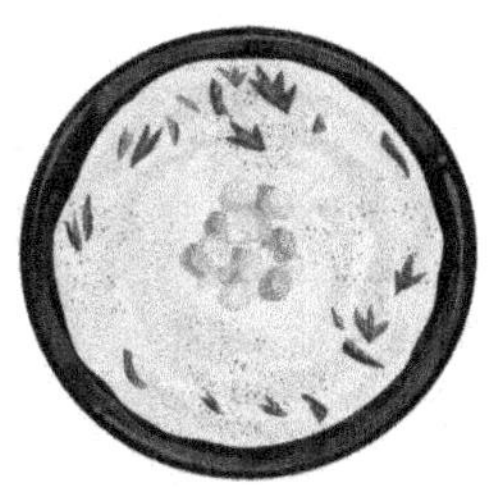

Lebanese Hummus

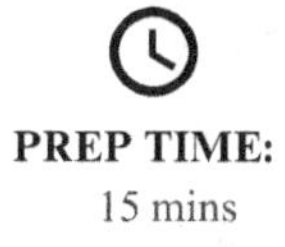 **PREP TIME:** 15 mins	 **COOK TIME:** 0 mins	 **SERVINGS:** 6	 **COURSE:** Lunch

Nutritional Value:	Calories: 152kcal	Fat: 15g	Carb: 5g	Protein: 2g

INGREDIENTS:

- 2-15 ounces cans chickpeas, drained and rinsed
- 2 cloves garlic, crushed
- 1/4 cup tahini paste
- 1/3 cup freshly squeezed lemon juice
- 1/4 cup extra virgin olive oil
- 1/4 tsp paprika
- 1/2 tsp salt
- 3 tbsp cold water
- pine nuts for garnish (optional)

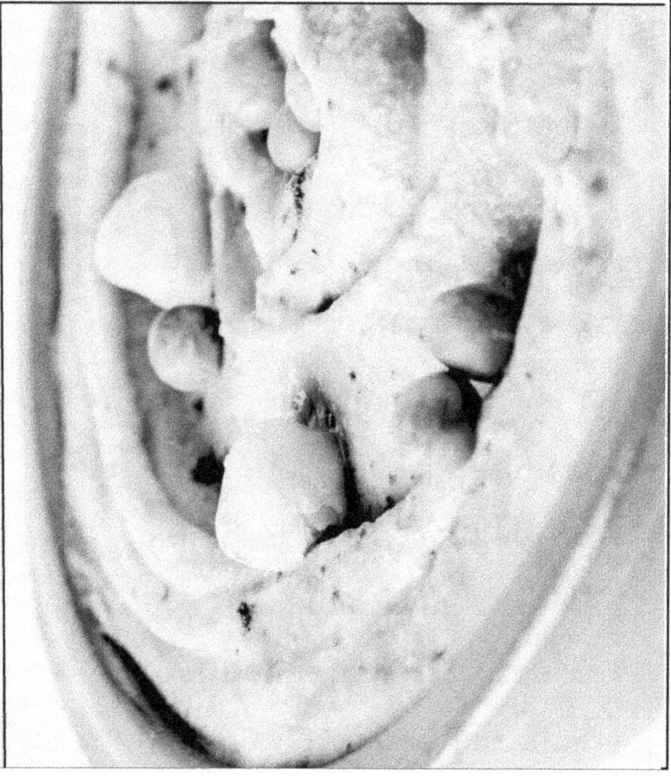

DIRECTIONS:

- To begin, chop the garlic in a food processor.
- Blend in the food processor the remaining ingredients until the desired consistency is reached.
- Blend in cold water to achieve a smoother consistency.

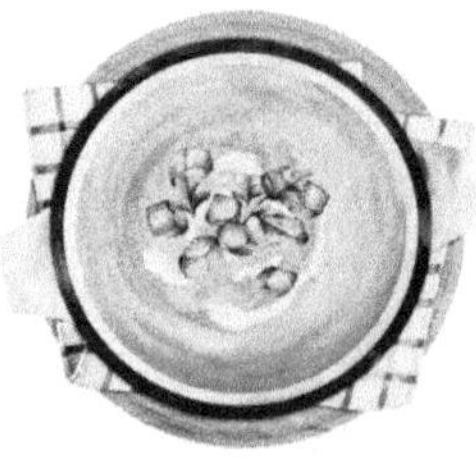

Garlic Soup with Egg and Croutons

			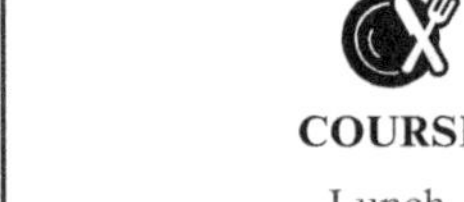
PREP TIME:	**COOK TIME:**	**SERVINGS:**	**COURSE:**
5 mins	35 mins	2	Lunch

Nutritional Value:	Calories: 473kcal	Fat: 35g	Carb: 24g	Protein: 19g

INGREDIENTS:

- 2 slices stale bread (you can toast the bread if not stale), cut into bite sized pieces
- 2 eggs
- 6 cloves garlic
- 1 tsp sweet paprika
- 1 liter chicken broth or vegetable broth homemade is best or store bought (low sodium)
- 1/4 cup extra virgin olive oil
- Salt and pepper, to taste (at least ½ teaspoon pepper)

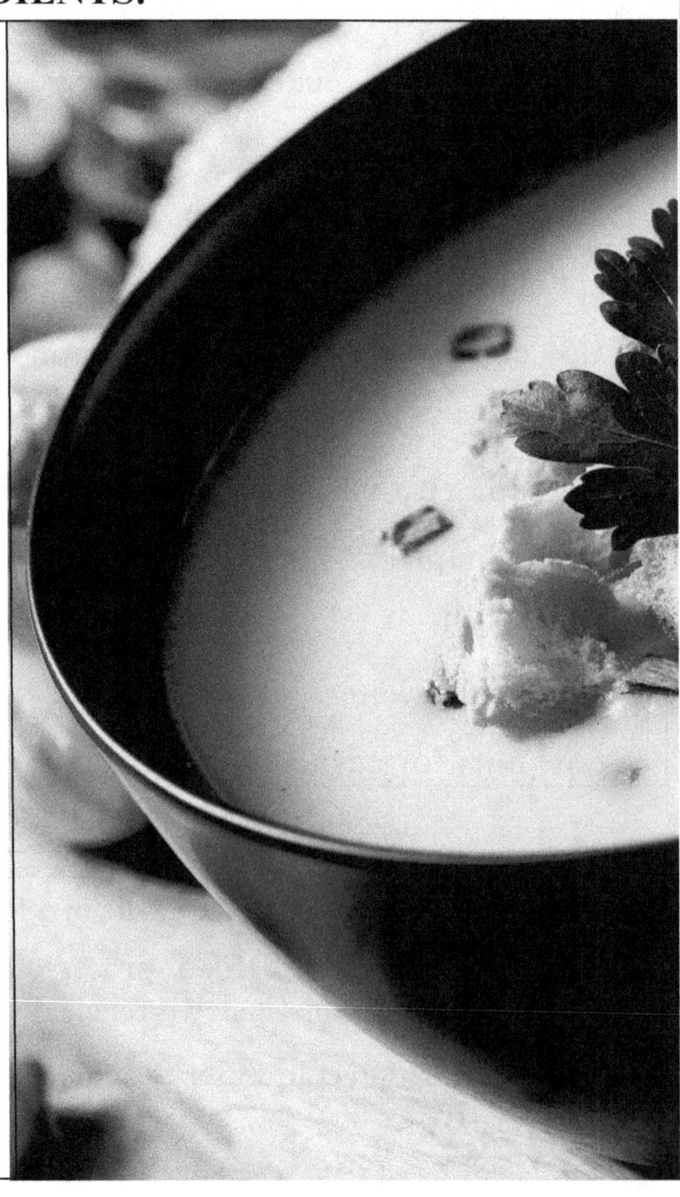

DIRECTIONS:

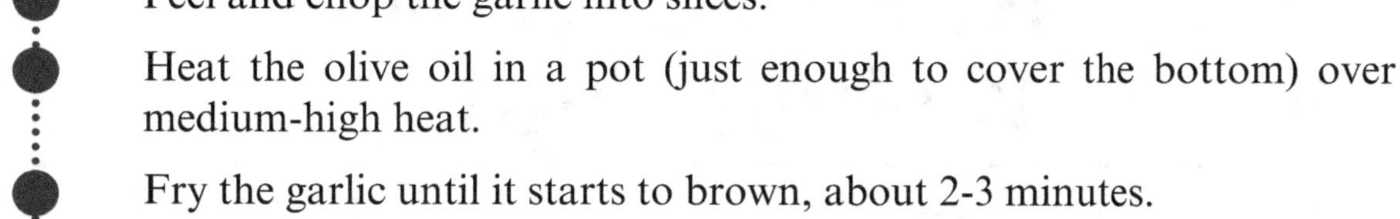

- Peel and chop the garlic into slices.

- Heat the olive oil in a pot (just enough to cover the bottom) over medium-high heat.

- Fry the garlic until it starts to brown, about 2-3 minutes.

- Add the bread to the pot and fry it with the garlic until it is soaked in the oil.

- Reduce the heat to low and stir in the paprika. Pour in the broth and whisk to combine.

- Bring the soup to a low boil, then reduce to a low simmer for 25 minutes. When the bread is soft and the soup has a rich brown color, it is done.

- Season with salt and pepper to taste, using at least 12 tsp pepper.

- Remove the soup from the heat and immediately crack the eggs within to cook in the residual heat. Incorporate the eggs into the soup. Warm food.

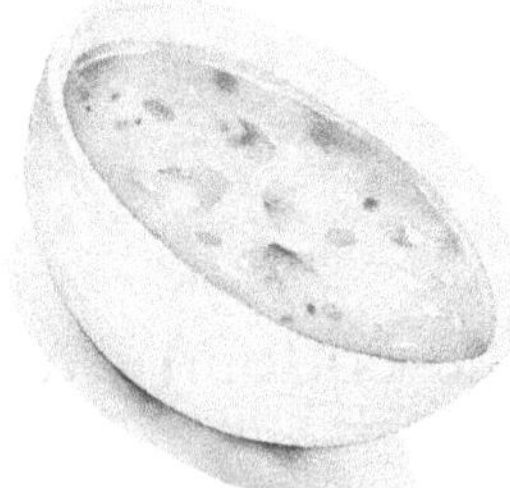

Muhammara (Roasted Red Pepper and Walnut Dip)

PREP TIME:
10 mins

COOK TIME:
20 mins

SERVINGS:
8

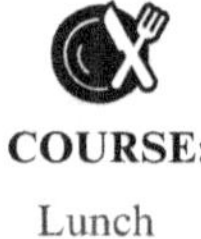

COURSE:
Lunch

Nutritional Value:	Calories: 174kcal	Fat: 17g	Carb: 6g	Protein: 3g

INGREDIENTS:

- 2 roasted red bell peppers
- 1 cup walnuts
- 2 cloves garlic
- 1 tsp pomegranate molasses
- 1/2 lemon juice
- 1 tsp cumin
- 1 pinch crushed red pepper flakes
- 1 tsp salt
- 1/4 cup extra virgin olive oil
- 1/4 cup breadcrumbs

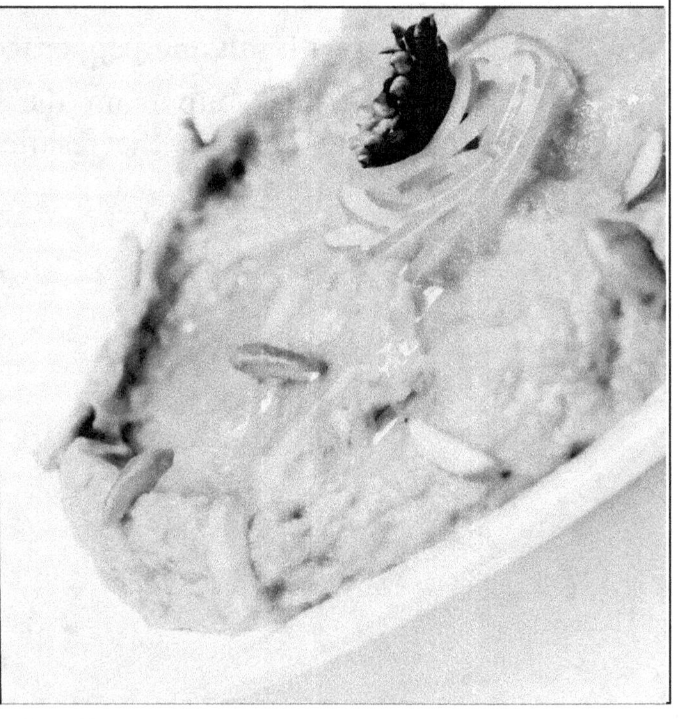

DIRECTIONS:

- Roast bell peppers in half and deseeded on a sheet pan for 20 minutes at 400 degrees. Flip midway through. To toast your walnuts at the same time, place them on a sheet pan and roast for about 10 minutes (keeping an eye on them so they don't burn).

- Blend the red peppers and walnuts with the remaining ingredients until smooth and creamy.

- Garnish with an olive oil drizzle, pomegranate molasses drizzle, and a sprinkle of crushed red or Aleppo pepper.

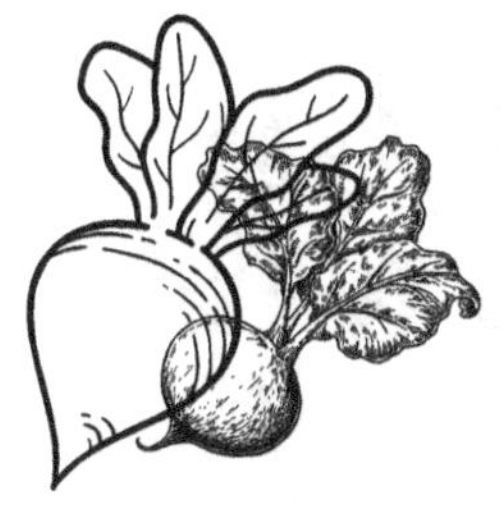

Beet and Carrot Salad with Walnuts and Goat Cheese

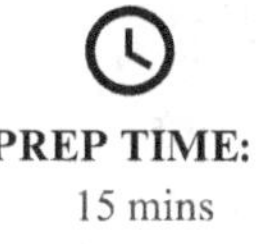 **PREP TIME:** 15 mins	 **COOK TIME:** 0 mins	 **SERVINGS:** 4	 **COURSE:** Lunch

Nutritional Value:	Calories: 275kcal	Fat: 16g	Carb: 27g	Protein: 10g

INGREDIENTS:

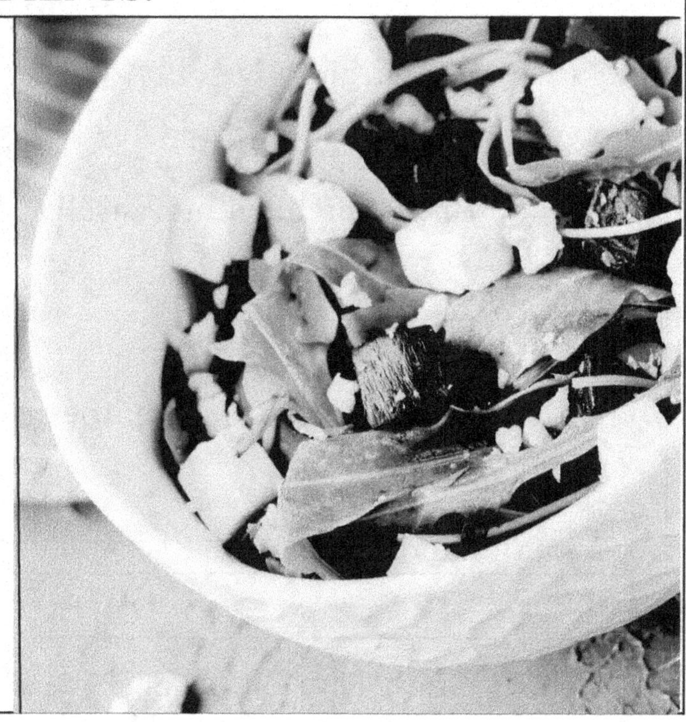

- 4 cups lettuce
- 2 carrots, peeled and shredded
- 1 large raw beets, peeled and shredded or 2 medium
- 1/4 red onion, sliced thin
- 1/4 cup dried cranberries
- 1/2 cup goat cheese, crumbled
- 1/2 cup walnuts
- 1/2 cup Dijon Vinaigrette see recipe

DIRECTIONS:

- Toast the walnuts
- Combine all ingredients in a large salad bowl. Serve

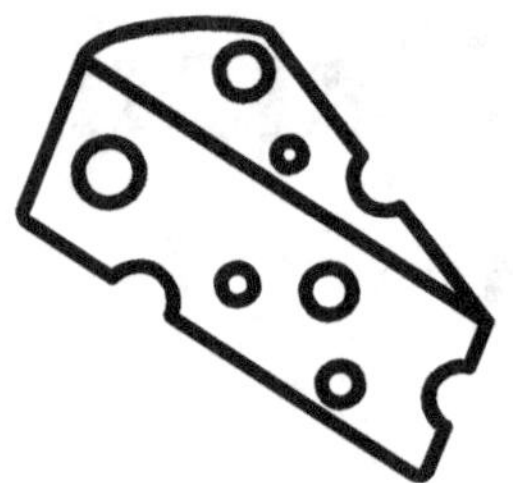

Grilled Cheese with Feta and Sun Dried Tomatoe

PREP TIME:
5 mins

COOK TIME:
10 mins

SERVINGS:
2

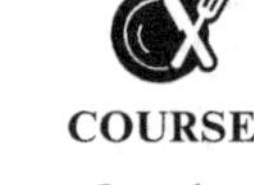

COURSE:
Lunch

Nutritional Value:	Calories: 514kcal	Fat: 35g	Carb: 33g	Protein: 19g

INGREDIENTS:

- 3 tbsp extra virgin olive oil
- 4 slices whole grain bread
- 1/2 cup finely shredded mozzarella cheese
- 1/3 cup feta cheese
- 1/4 cup sun-dried tomatoes, chopped
- 2 small handful arugula

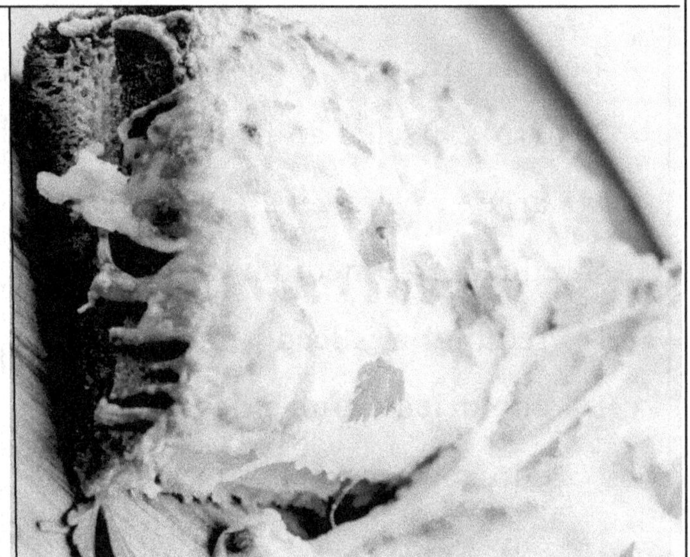

DIRECTIONS:

- Brush olive oil on one side of each slice of bread (using all three tablespoons of oil). Place each slice of bread, oil side down, on a baking sheet.

- Place half of the mozzarella, half of the feta (slightly crumbled), half of the tomatoes, and half of the arugula on one slice of bread. Wrap in a slice of bread. Make the second sandwich in the same manner.

- Preheat a nonstick or cast iron skillet over medium heat. Cook the sandwiches on one side until golden brown (approximately 4-5 minutes). Cook till golden brown on the second side. Consume quickly!

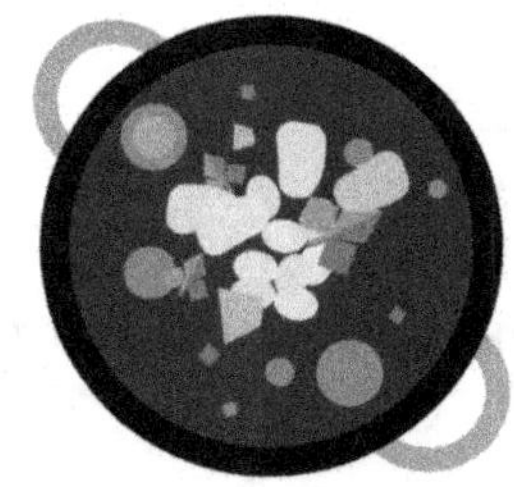

Moroccan Harira (Lentil and Chickpea Soup)

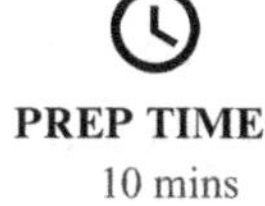 **PREP TIME:** 10 mins	 **COOK TIME:** 30 mins	 **SERVINGS:** 6	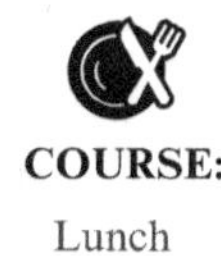 **COURSE:** Lunch

Nutritional Value:

Calories: 194kcal	Fat: 6g	Carb: 28g	Protein: 8g

INGREDIENTS:

- 1 large onion
- 1/2 bunch cilantro (about a cup, loosely packed), washed, large stems removed
- 1/2 bunch parsley (about a cup, loosely packed), washed, large stems removed
- 1 stick celery, coarsely chopped
- 4 tomatoes, skins removed
- 1/2 cup dry green lentils, rinsed and checked for stones
- 1 tsp salt
- 1 tsp ground pepper
- 1 tsp turmeric
- 1/2 tsp ginger
- 1/2 piece any salted vegetable bullion cube
- 2 tbsp extra virgin olive oil
- 4 tbsp tomato paste
- 1 cup cooked (canned) chickpeas
- 1/2 cup (2 ounces) thin pasta (angel hair), broken in quarters
- 2 tbsp all purpose white flour

DIRECTIONS:

- In a blender or food processor, combine the onion, half of the cilantro, half of the parsley, celery, and tomatoes. Blend until completely smooth.

- In a large soup saucepan, combine the blended vegetables and 2 cups of water. Bring the lentils, salt, pepper, turmeric, ginger, bouillon cube, olive oil, and tomato paste to a boil over high heat. Bring to a boil again, then reduce to a low heat for 10 minutes.

- Add chickpeas, pasta, and 4 cups water after 10 minutes. Bring to a boil and reduce to a low heat for 5 minutes while you prepare the flour/water mixture.

- 1/4 cup flour and 1/4 cup water, combined in a blender or food processor, until smooth. Stir the flour-water mixture into the soup slowly. Simmer for 5 minutes more.

- Simmer for a few minutes after adding the rest of the chopped herbs. Season with salt and pepper to taste.

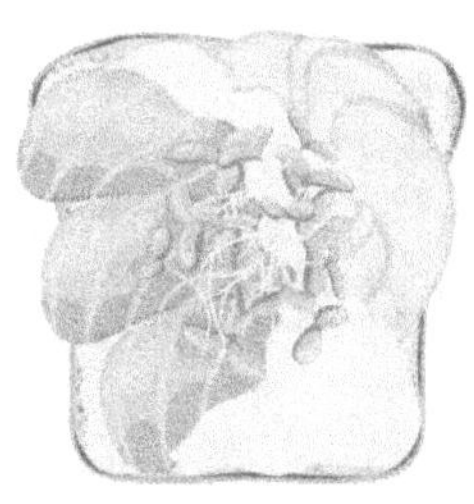

Avocado Toast with Smoked Salmon, Fresh Dill and Capers

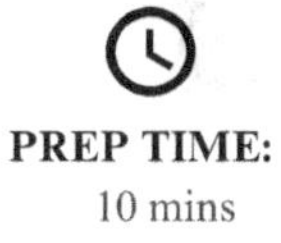

PREP TIME:
10 mins

COOK TIME:
0 mins

SERVINGS:
2

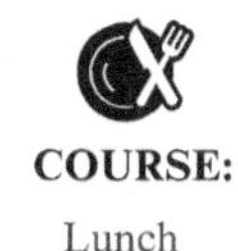

COURSE:
Lunch

Nutritional Value:	Calories: 199kcal	Fat: 16g	Carb: 10g	Protein: 7g

INGREDIENTS:

- 1 ripe avocado
- 1/2 lemon juice
- Dash of salt
- 2 ounces smoked salmon, thinly sliced
- A few small stems fresh dill
- 10 capers
- A few thin slices of red onion
- 2 large slices bread or 4 small slices of bread

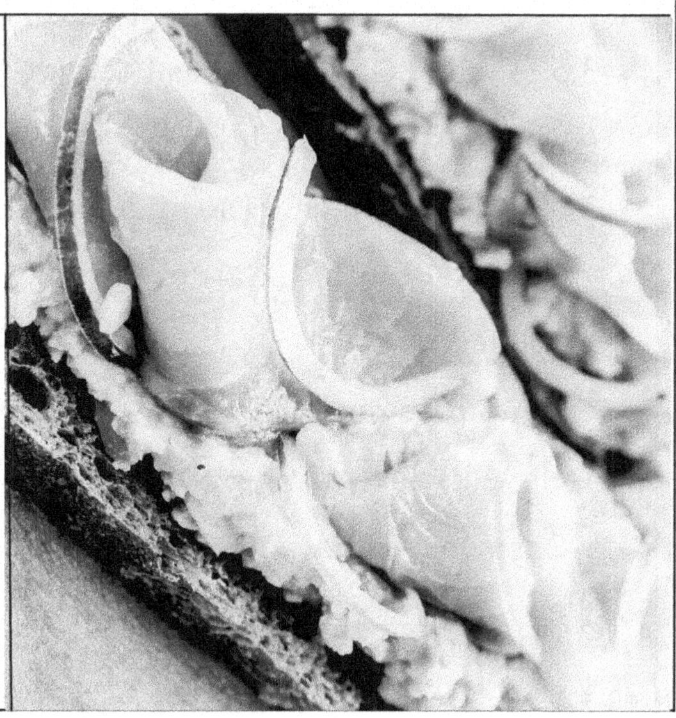

DIRECTIONS:

- Cut the avocado in half and remove the pit. Scoop out the flesh and mash it with a little salt and lemon juice.
- Toast the bread. On toast, spread avocado. Finish with capers.
- Top the avocado and capers with a few slices of smoked salmon, followed by dill and red onion slices. Serve right away.

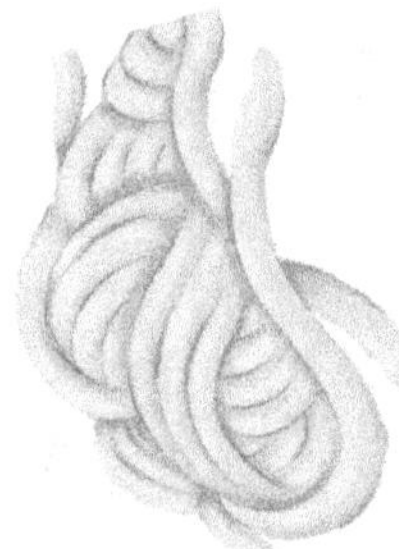

Pasta Genovese in Pasta or Potato Salad or on Bread

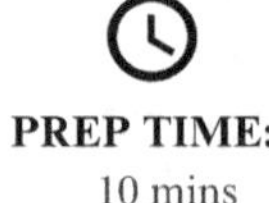 **PREP TIME:** 10 mins	 **COOK TIME:** 0 mins	 **SERVINGS:** 8	 **COURSE:** Lunch

Nutritional Value:	Calories: 222kcal	Fat: 22g	Carb: 2g	Protein: 7g

INGREDIENTS:

- 3.5 ounces Genovese basil leaves (sweet basil) by weight
- 1 cup Parmesan cheese, shredded
- 1/4 cup Pecorino Sardo cheese, shredded
- 1/3 cup pine nuts
- 1 clove garlic
- 1/2 tsp coarse sea salt
- 1/2 cup extra virgin olive oil (plus 1 tbsp to add on top)

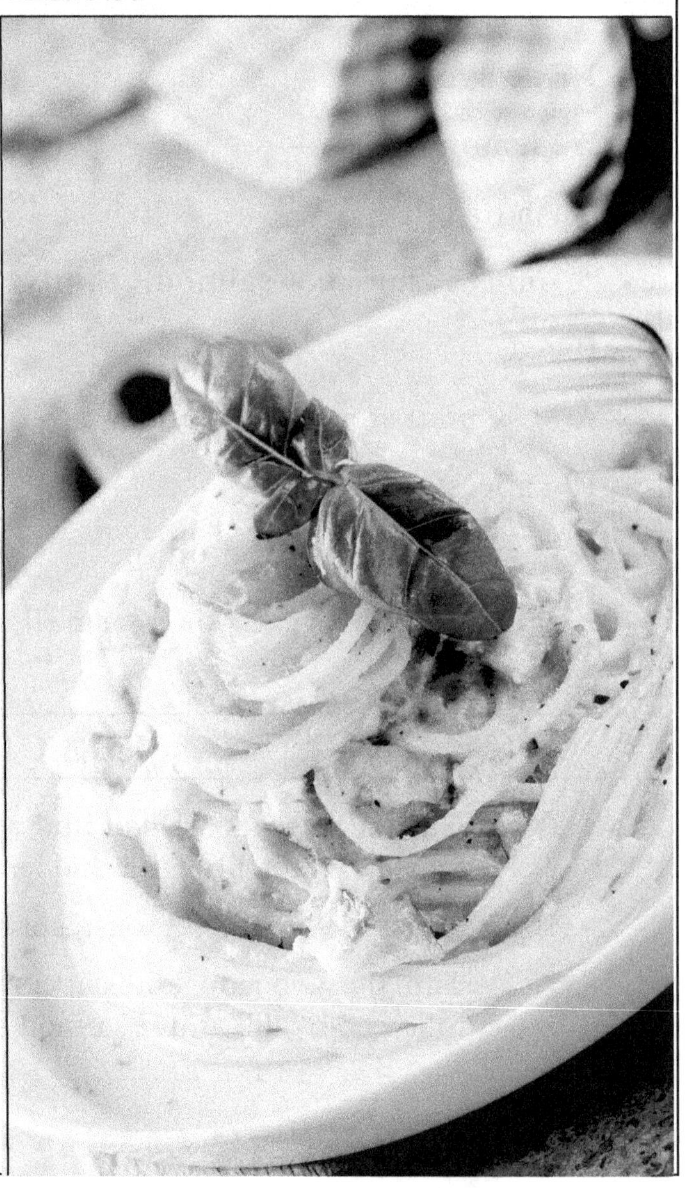

DIRECTIONS:

- Wash basil leaves gently in cold water and then drain until completely dry.

- Blend Parmesan cheese, Pecorino Sardo cheese, pine nuts, and garlic in a food processor.

- Season with basil leaves and salt.

- Continue to combine until the mixture is smooth, slowly sprinkling the olive oil on top of the other ingredients as you go. If you over-blend the sauce, the blades will begin to burn the basil.

- Finally, pour the pesto into a jar and cover with extra olive oil to prevent oxidation.

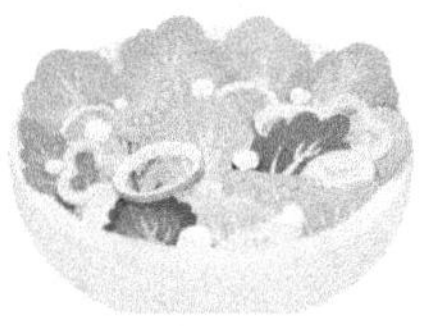

Authentic Greek Salad

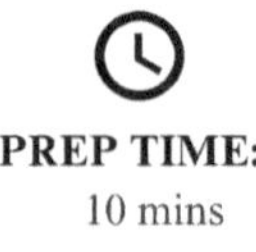 **PREP TIME:** 10 mins	 **COOK TIME:** 0 mins	 **SERVINGS:** 4	 **COURSE:** Lunch

Nutritional Value:	Calories: 469kcal	Fat: 43g	Carb: 14g	Protein: 11g

INGREDIENTS:

- 1 pint cherry tomatoes
- 2 large cucumbers, peeled and sliced
- 1/4 red onion, cut into thin strips
- 1 red bell pepper, cut into thin strips
- 20 kalamata olives
- 8 ounces feta cheese
- 1/2 cup extra virgin olive oil
- 2 tbsp red wine vinegar or lemon juice
- 1 tsp oregano
- salt and pepper, to taste

DIRECTIONS:

- In a mixing bowl, combine all of the vegetables and olives.

- Add feta cheese, olive oil, lemon juice (or vinegar), and oregano to taste. Season with salt and pepper to taste.

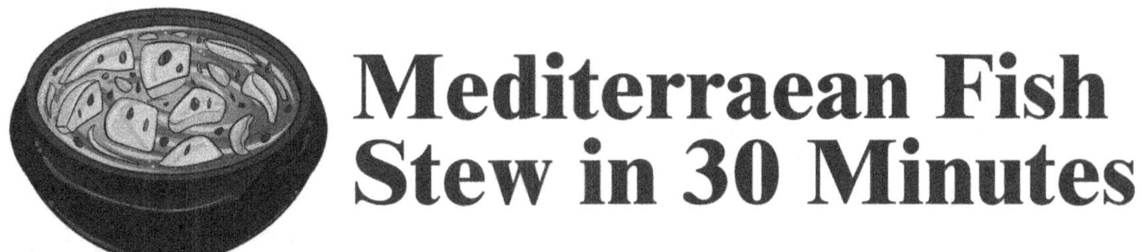

Mediterraean Fish Stew in 30 Minutes

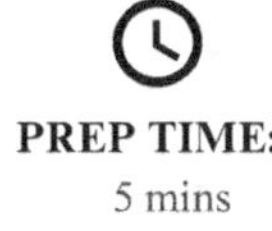

PREP TIME:
5 mins

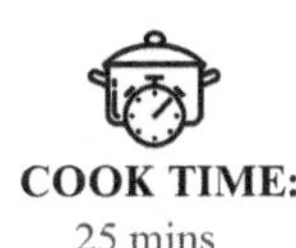

COOK TIME:
25 mins

SERVINGS:
4

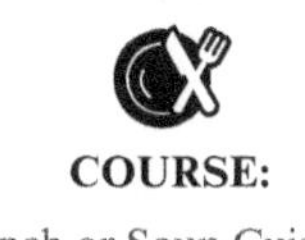

COURSE:
Lunch or Soup Cuisine

Nutritional Value:	Calories: 391kcal	Fat: 15g	Carb: 36g	Protein: 29g

INGREDIENTS:

- 2 tbsp butter
- 2 tbsp extra virgin olive oil
- 1 onion, chopped
- 1 carrot, sliced into thin rounds
- 1 tbsp flour
- 3 medium potatoes, peeled and cut into bite sized cubes
- 1 pound white fish (cod, halibut, haddock) boneless
- 4 cups chicken broth, low sodium or regular
- 1/2 tsp smoked paprika
- Salt and pepper, to taste

DIRECTIONS:

- In a heavy-bottomed pot, melt the butter and olive oil. Cook until the onions and carrots are tender (approximately 3 minutes). Stir in the flour, followed by the potatoes. Cook for 1 minute on medium heat.

- Bring the chicken broth to a boil. Mix in the fish and smoked paprika. Cover and cook for 15- 20 minutes, stirring periodically, until the potatoes are tender. Flake the fish into small pieces.

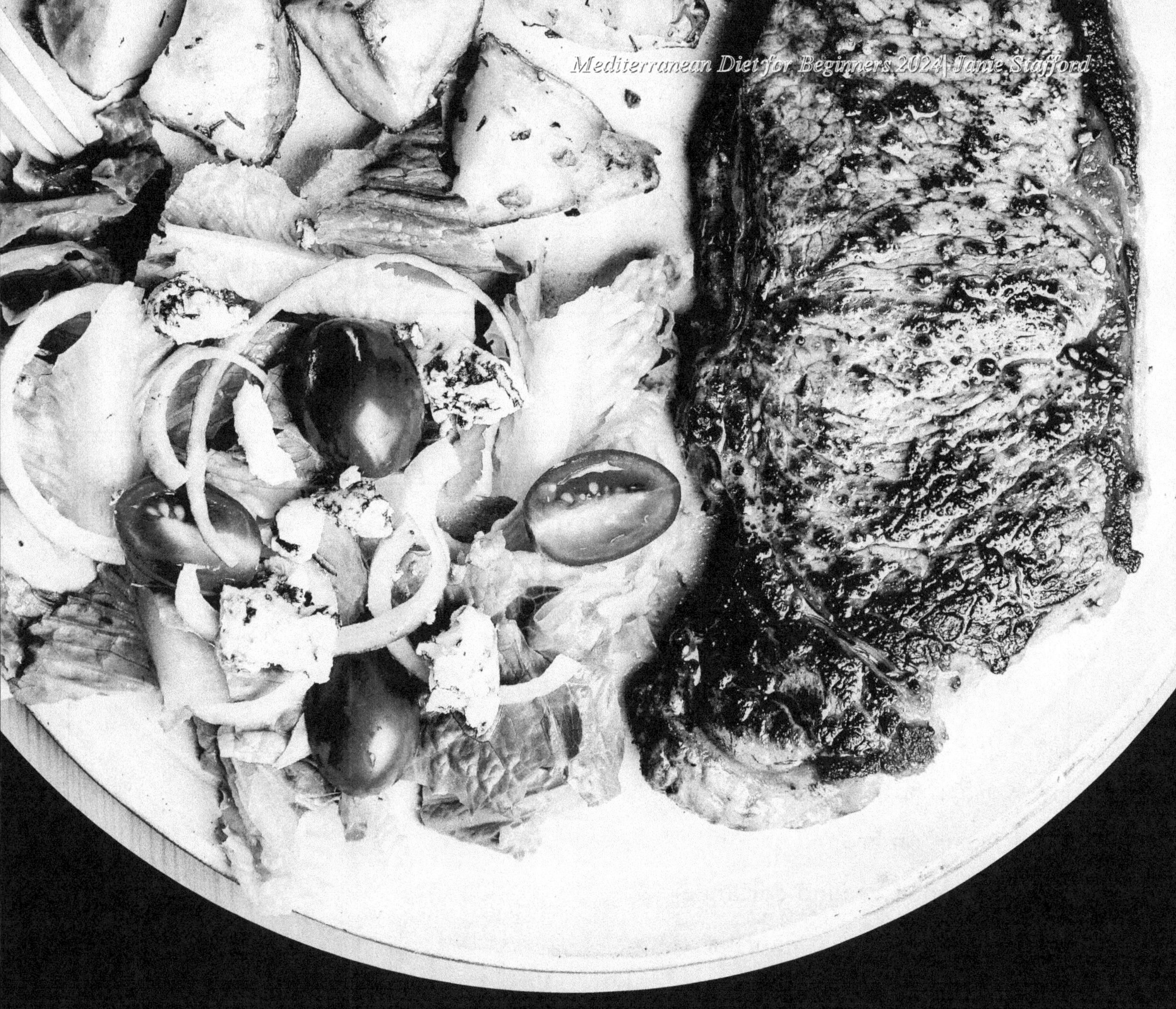

DINNER
RECIPES

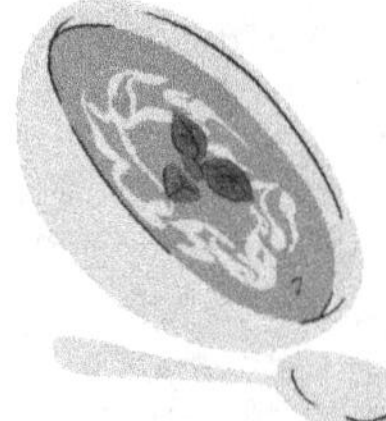

Garlicky Spinach and Chickpea Soup with Lemon and Pecorino Romano

 **PREP TIME:** 10 mins	 **COOK TIME:** 40 mins	 **SERVINGS:** 4	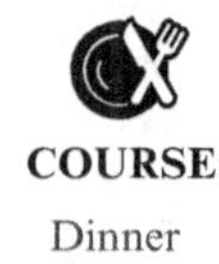 **COURSE:** Dinner

Nutritional Value:	Calories: 468kcal	Fat: 18g	Carb: 58g	Protein: 22g

INGREDIENTS:

- Two 15-ounce cans chickpeas
- Extra-virgin olive oil
- 1 large yellow onion, roughly chopped
- 4 or 5 large garlic cloves, minced
- Kosher salt
- 1 teaspoon ground cumin
- 1 teaspoon ground coriander
- ¾ teaspoon sweet paprika
- ½ teaspoon crushed red pepper flakes
- ½ teaspoon freshly ground black pepper
- 4 cups vegetable stock or low-sodium chicken broth
- 2 cups (packed) fresh baby spinach (2 to 3 ounces)
- ½ cup roughly chopped fresh flat-leaf parsley
- 1 large lemon, cut in half
- ½ cup grated Pecorino Romano cheese
- Crusty bread, for serving

DIRECTIONS:

- Drain the chickpeas, reserving ½ cup of their liquid.

- In a big pot, heat 3 tablespoons of olive oil over medium heat until it starts to shimmer. Throw in the onion and garlic and season with a generous pinch of salt.

- Heat a pot over medium heat and add about ½ teaspoon of oil. Cook, stirring regularly, until fragrant, about 5 minutes. Add the cumin, coriander, paprika, red pepper flakes and black pepper and cook, stirring regularly for about 30 seconds.

- Add the chickpeas and stir to coat with the spices. Using a potato masher or the back of a sturdy fork, roughly mash the chickpeas (you're just looking to break some of them up).

- Pour in the stock and the reserved chickpea liquid. Increase the heat and bring to a boil, then boil for 5 minutes. Reduce the heat to medium-low and partly cover the pot with the lid. Simmer the chickpeas for 30 minutes.

- Turn off the heat. Stir in the spinach and parsley, and let the soup sit for 1 minute, until the spinach wilts. Squeeze half a lemon over the soup, stir and taste, adding more lemon juice to your liking.

- Divide the soup into serving bowls and top each bowl with a drizzle of olive oil and a bit of grated Pecorino Romano cheese. Serve with crusty bread.

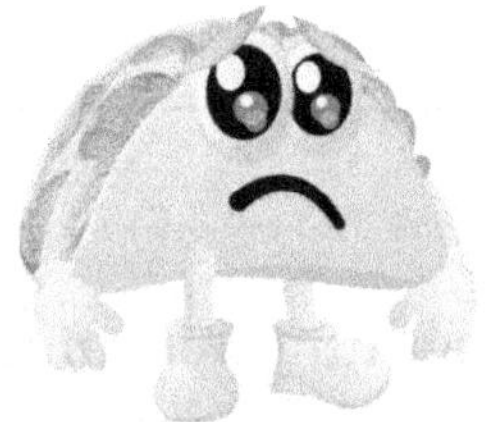

Spicy Sweet Potato Tacos

PREP TIME:
10 mins

COOK TIME:
10mins

SERVINGS:
4

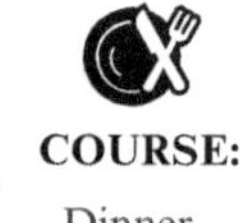
COURSE:
Dinner

Nutritional Value:	Calories: 204kcal	Fat: 3g	Carb: 41g	Protein: 5g

INGREDIENTS:

- Extra-virgin olive oil, as needed
- 1 small onion, chopped
- 2 garlic cloves, chopped
- Kosher salt and freshly ground black pepper, to taste2 or 3 medium sweet potatoes, washed
- 3 teaspoons chili powder
- 1 teaspoon ground cumin
- ½ teaspoon crushed red pepper flakes
- Corn tortillas, fresh cilantro, limes, avocado and pickled onions, for serving

DIRECTIONS:

- Grate the sweet potatoes using a box grater (no need to skin them). A food processor with a grater attachment can also be used.

- Meanwhile, in a medium skillet over medium heat, heat the olive oil. Cook until the onion and garlic are aromatic and starting to soften, about 3 minutes. Season with salt and pepper to taste. Cook until the sweet potato is tender, 5 to 7 minutes, after adding the chili powder, cumin, and red pepper flakes.

- Fill warm corn tortillas with the filling and top with fresh lime juice, cilantro, avocado, and pickled onions.

Chickpea Caesar Salad with a Cheater's Dressing

 **PREP TIME:** 15 mins	 **COOK TIME:** 15 mins	 **SERVINGS:** 4	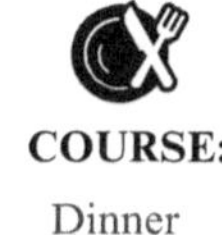 **COURSE:** Dinner

Nutritional Value:	Calories: 557kcal	Fat: 39g	Carb: 40g	Protein: 15g

INGREDIENTS:

CRISPY CHICKPEAS

- One 15-ounce can chickpeas, rinsed and drained
- Extra-virgin olive oil
- ½ teaspoon smoked paprika
- ½ teaspoon kosher salt

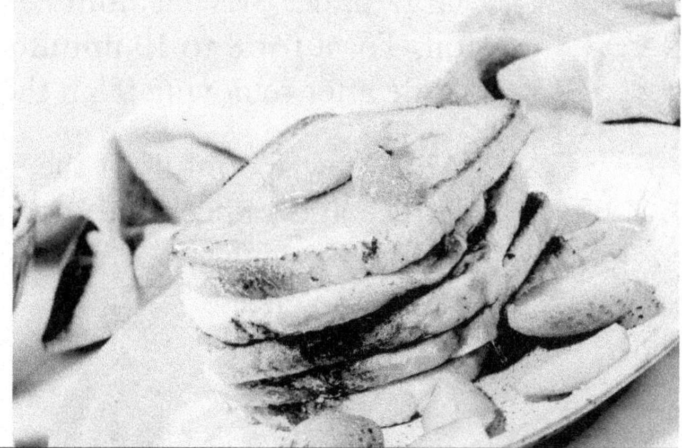

CHEATER'S CAESAR DRESSING

- ½ cup mayonnaise
- Juice of ½ lemon (about 2 tablespoons)
- ¼ cup finely grated Parmesan cheese
- 2 teaspoons Dijon mustard
- 1 garlic clove, grated
- ½ teaspoon Worcestershire sauce

ASSEMBLY

- Extra-virgin olive oil
- 2 cups cubed bread (such as sourdough)
- Kosher salt
- 1 head romaine, chopped or torn into bite-size pieces
- ½ head radicchio, cored and chopped into bite-size pieces
- Grated Parmesan cheese, to serve

DIRECTIONS:

HOW TO MAKE THE CRISPY CHICKPEAS: Preheat the oven to 425 degrees Fahrenheit. Toss the chickpeas with a couple tablespoons of olive oil, paprika, and salt on a baking sheet until coated. Bake for 15 to 20 minutes, or until the chickpeas are brown and crisp.

MAKE THE DRESSING: In a small mixing bowl, combine the mayonnaise, lemon juice, Parmesan, mustard, garlic, and Worcestershire. Season with salt and pepper to taste. If the dressing appears excessively thick (it should be the consistency of heavy cream), whisk in a teaspoon of water. The dressing can be made up to 1 day ahead of time and refrigerated.

ASSEMBLE THE SALAD: Heat a few tablespoons of olive oil in a large skillet over medium heat. Toss in the cubed bread to coat in the oil. Toast for 8 to 10 minutes, or until golden brown on all sides. Set aside after removing from the heat and seasoning with salt.

Add a few spoonfuls of the dressing to a large salad bowl. Toss in the lettuce and radicchio to coat, adding additional dressing if required. Before serving, top with crispy chickpeas, croutons, and extra Parmesan cheese.

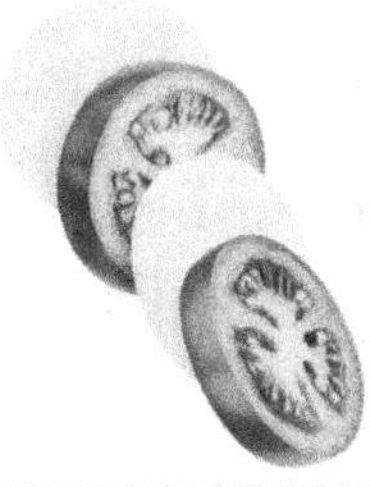

Marinated White Bean and Tomato Salad

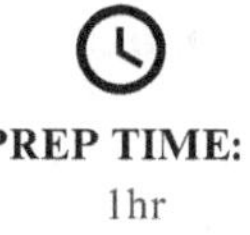 **PREP TIME:** 1hr	 **COOK TIME:** 1hr	 **SERVINGS:** 4 to 6 servings	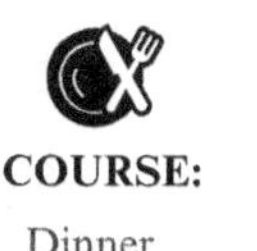 **COURSE:** Dinner

Nutritional Value:	Calories: 426kcal	Fat: 22g	Carb: 45g	Protein: 14g

INGREDIENTS:

- ½ cup extra-virgin olive oil
- 4 garlic cloves, thinly sliced
- Two 15.5-ounce cans white beans, such as butter beans or cannellini, drained and rinsed
- Zest of 1 lemon, finely grated
- 2 sprigs oregano, leaves removed (about 1 tablespoon fresh oregano leaves, or 2
- tablespoons dried oregano)
- Kosher salt
- 2 pints cherry tomatoes or a couple large heirloom tomatoes, or a mix of shapes and sizes

DIRECTIONS:

- Heat the oil and garlic in a small saucepan or skillet over medium-low heat until the garlic is just starting to turn golden brown and smells aromatic, about 5 minutes.

- Place the drained beans in a large mixing basin or resealable container, then drizzle with the hot garlic oil and toss to incorporate.

- Season with salt to taste after adding the lemon zest and oregano. Allow to settle at room temperature for at least 1 hour, or seal and refrigerate overnight. Remove from the fridge about 1 hour before serving to bring to room temperature so the oil does not become cold and congealed.

- Half the cherry tomatoes (or cut the heirlooms into big bite-size pieces or wedges) 30 minutes or 1 hour before serving and season liberally with salt. Please do not skip this step as it helps to accentuate the tomato flavor.

- Allow them to sit separately from the beans until just before serving, then remove the tomatoes (leaving the juices behind) and mix them into the beans. Seasoning should be tasted and adjusted as needed. If you want to brighten it up, add a dash of sherry or red wine vinegar, as well as some fresh oregano leaves. If you want to add some heat, add some crushed red pepper flakes. Place on a serving plate.

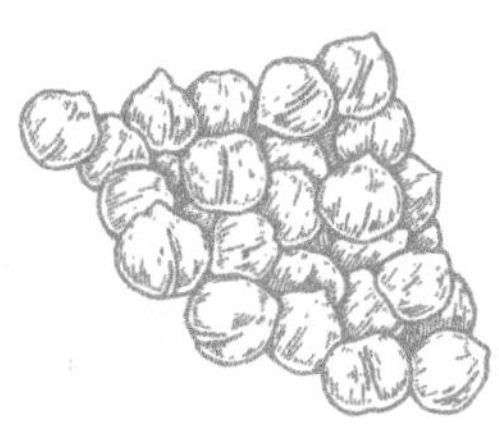

Crispy Chickpeas and Scallops with Garlic-Harissa Oil

 **PREP TIME:** 5 mins	 **COOK TIME:** 20 mins	 **SERVINGS:** 2 to 3 servings	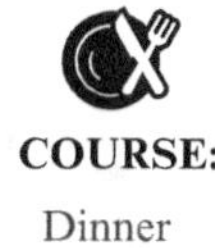 **COURSE:** Dinner

Nutritional Value:	Calories: 461kcal	Fat: 31g	Carb: 27g	Protein: 21g

INGREDIENTS:

- 12 ounces wild-caught sea scallops (thawed, if frozen), side muscles removed
- Kosher salt and ground black pepper
- Extra-virgin olive oil
- One 15-ounce can of chickpeas, drained and rinsed
- 2 scallions, trimmed, whites and greens separated and chopped
- ¾ teaspoon sumac
- ½ teaspoon ground cumin
- 2 medium garlic cloves, thinly sliced
- 3 to 4 tablespoons high-quality store-bought harissa
- 1 large lemon, cut in half

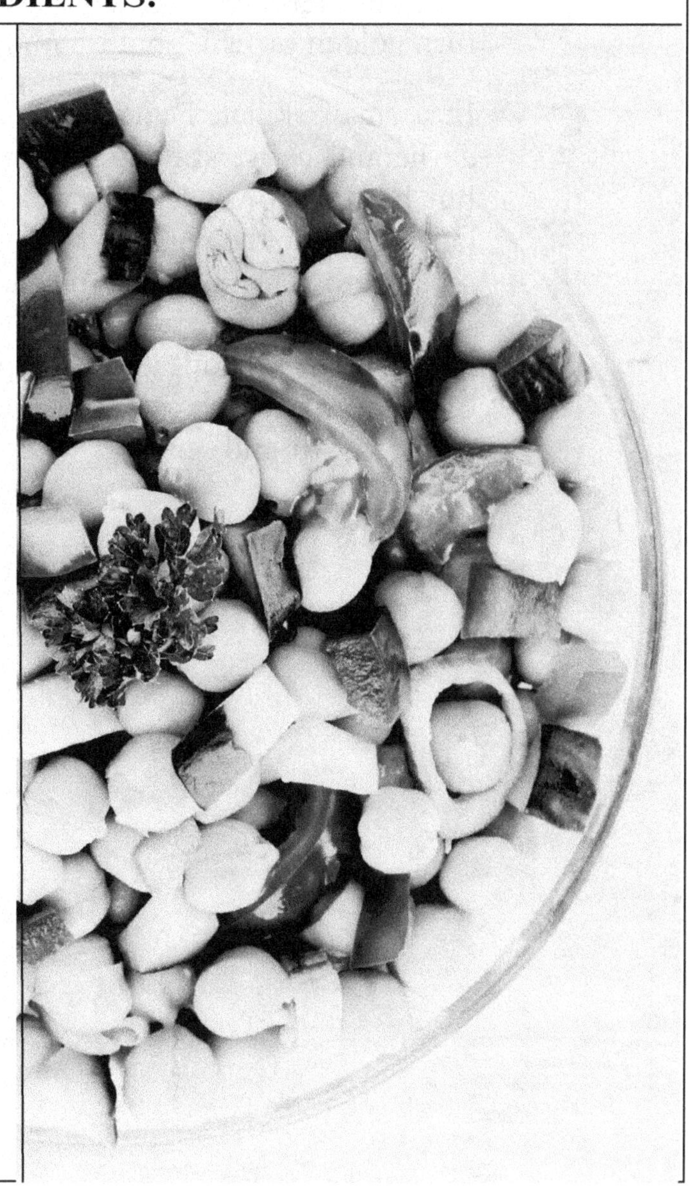

DIRECTIONS:

Using paper towels, pat the scallops dry and season them generously with salt and pepper. Heat 2 tablespoons of olive oil in a large cast iron skillet over medium-high heat until shimmering.

Place the scallops in the pan in a single layer, making sure the first scallop sizzles immediately on contact. Cook the scallops for 2 minutes on each side, flipping them over only once, until golden brown. If the scallop does not release easily from the skillet, wait a few more seconds. Place the scallops on a plate.

Add another tablespoon of olive oil to the skillet and add the chickpeas and the white parts of the scallions. Season with the sumac, cumin, salt and black pepper (about ½ teaspoon each). Cook over medium-high heat, tossing occasionally, until the chickpeas crisp and turn golden brown, about 5 minutes.

In a small skillet, heat ¼ cup olive oil over medium heat. Add the garlic and cook, stirring frequently, until it barely gains some color but hasn't browned. Remove the pan from the heat and stir in the harissa. Place the scallops back in the large skillet and give them a few seconds to warm up with the chickpeas.

Transfer the scallops and chickpeas to a platter, squeeze the lemon all over, then add the scallion greens. Spoon the garlic and harissa oil over top, stir and serve.

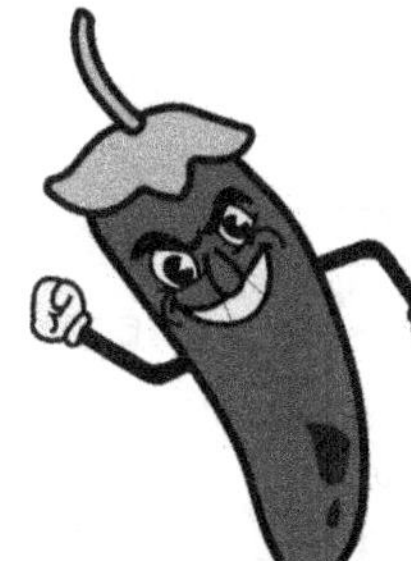

Mediterranean Quinoa Bowls with Roasted Red Pepper Sauce

 **PREP TIME:** 15mins	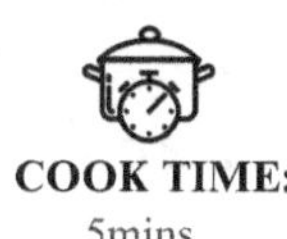 **COOK TIME:** 5mins	 **SERVINGS:** 8	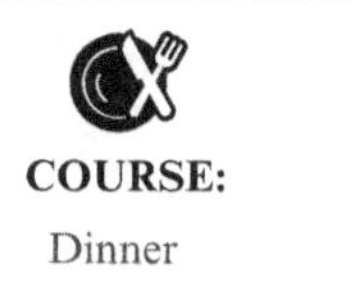 **COURSE:** Dinner

Nutritional Value:	Calories: 381kcal	Fat: 25.6g	Carb: 30.9g	Protein: 10.9g

INGREDIENTS:

Roasted Red Pepper Sauce:

- 1 16 ounce jar roasted red peppers, drained (or roast your own red peppers and win the
- food game!)
- 1 clove garlic
- 1/2 teaspoon salt (more to taste)
- juice of one lemon
- 1/2 cup olive oil
- 1/2 cup almonds

For the Mediterranean Bowls (build your own bowls based on what you like)

- cooked quinoa
- spinach, kale, or cucumber
- feta cheese
- kalamata olives
- pepperoncini
- thinly sliced red onion
- hummus
- fresh basil or parsley
- olive oil, lemon juice, salt, pepper

DIRECTIONS:

- In a food processor or blender, combine all of the sauce ingredients and pulse until almost smooth. The texture should be thick and textured.

- Cook the quinoa according to package directions (I always do mine in a rice cooker while I prepare the rest of the ingredients). When the quinoa is finished, assemble a Mediterranean Quinoa Bowl!

- Store leftovers in separate containers and assemble each bowl just before serving, particularly the greens and sauces, which may become mushy if stored with the rest of the ingredients.

NOTES:

- For a vegan-friendly option, substitute the feta cheese with white beans.

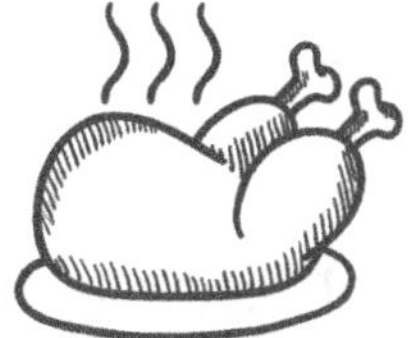 # Baked Chicken and Ricotta Meatballs

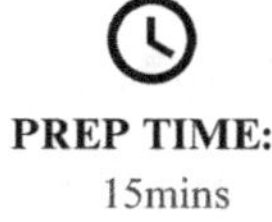 PREP TIME: 15mins	 COOK TIME: 15mins	 SERVINGS: 4	 COURSE: Dinner

Nutritional Value:	Calories: 454kcal	Fat: 27g	Carb: 20g	Protein: 36g

INGREDIENTS:

- 14 ounces (400g) broccolini, rough stems trimmed and thick pieces cut lengthwise
- 1 lemon, ends trimmed and thinly sliced
- 4 tablespoons extra-virgin olive oil, divided
- Kosher salt and freshly ground black pepper
- ½ teaspoon crushed red pepper flakes, or more if desired
- 1 large egg
- 2 garlic cloves, grated
- ¾ cup ricotta cheese, drained and lightly salted
- ½ cup parsley leaves and fine stems, roughly chopped
- ¾ cup panko breadcrumbs
- 1 pound ground chicken, preferably dark meat
- Juice of 1 lemon
- Grated Parmesan, for sprinkling (optional)

DIRECTIONS:

Preheat the oven to 425 degrees Fahrenheit.

Toss the broccoli and lemon slices with 3 tablespoons olive oil, salt, pepper, and red pepper flakes on a baking sheet. Set aside on a baking pan to cool while you create the meatballs.

MAKE THE MEATBALLS: In a medium mixing bowl, combine the egg, garlic, ricotta, 1 teaspoon salt, parsley, pepper, the remaining oil, breadcrumbs, and meat, and gently incorporate (too much mushing will result in tough and dry meatballs).

The meat should still be visible through the seasonings. Roll the beef into twenty loose—not tightly packed—rounds, somewhat smaller than golf balls, using a gentle rolling motion between your hands (the water will keep them from sticking to your palms). Place large pieces of baking paper on the counter to make cleanup easy.

Place the meatballs between the broccoli and lemon on the baking sheet. Bake for 15 to 20 minutes, or until the meatballs are browned and cooked through and the broccoli is crisp, shaking the baking sheet to move the meatballs and turning the tray over halfway to ensure equal cooking.

Remove from the oven, drizzle with lemon juice, and distribute among plates. If using, top with grated Parmesan.

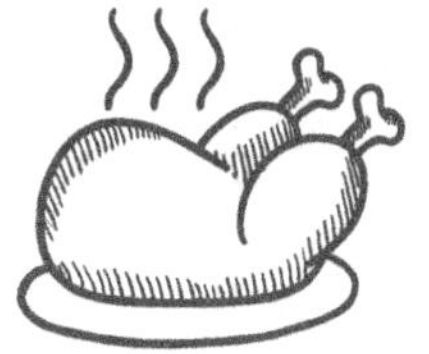

Winter One-Pan Chicken and Veggies

PREP TIME: 30mins	**COOK TIME:** 30mins	**SERVINGS:** 1/4 of batch	**COURSE:** Dinner

Nutritional Value:	Calories: 383.51kcal	Fat: 14.96g	Carb: 29.85g	Protein: 31.16g

INGREDIENTS:

- 2 tablespoons olive oil (divided)
- 3 cups baby potatoes (quartered)
- salt and pepper
- 1 bunch asparagus (trimmed and cut into bite-sized pieces)
- ½ zucchini (cut into bite-sized pieces)
- 1 tablespoon arrowroot starch (corn starch or all-purpose flour may be used)
- 1 lb boneless skinless chicken breast (roughly 2 large chicken breasts; cut into 1-inch cubes)
- 1 cup chicken stock
- ¼ cup balsamic vinegar
- ¼ teaspoon salt

To Serve

- ½ cup feta cheese crumbled
- ¼ cup pomegranate arils

DIRECTIONS:

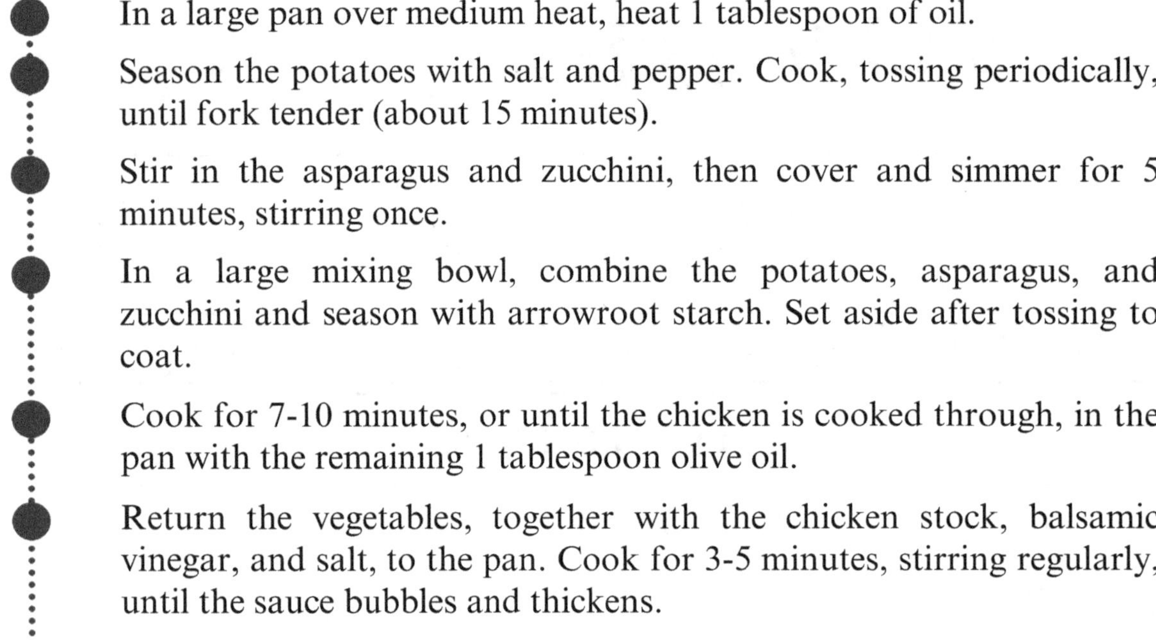

- In a large pan over medium heat, heat 1 tablespoon of oil.

- Season the potatoes with salt and pepper. Cook, tossing periodically, until fork tender (about 15 minutes).

- Stir in the asparagus and zucchini, then cover and simmer for 5 minutes, stirring once.

- In a large mixing bowl, combine the potatoes, asparagus, and zucchini and season with arrowroot starch. Set aside after tossing to coat.

- Cook for 7-10 minutes, or until the chicken is cooked through, in the pan with the remaining 1 tablespoon olive oil.

- Return the vegetables, together with the chicken stock, balsamic vinegar, and salt, to the pan. Cook for 3-5 minutes, stirring regularly, until the sauce bubbles and thickens.

- Serve immediately topped with pomegranates and feta.

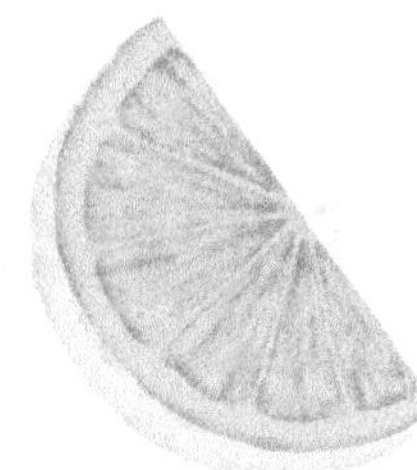

Lemon Salmon with Garlic and Thyme

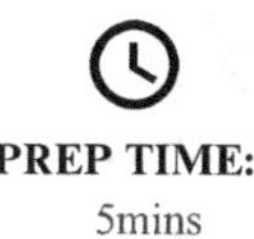			
PREP TIME: 5mins	**COOK TIME:** 5mins	**SERVINGS:** 4	**COURSE:** Dinner

Nutritional Value:	Calories: 356kcal	Fat: 23g	Carb: 3g	Protein: 32g

INGREDIENTS:

- Four 5- to 6-ounce salmon fillets
- Extra virgin olive oil, as needed
- Kosher salt and freshly ground black pepper
- 1 whole lemon, zested and sliced into thin rounds
- ½ teaspoon dried thyme
- 4 to 5 five garlic cloves, peeled and lightly crushed

DIRECTIONS:

- Preheat the oven to 400 degrees Fahrenheit.
- Place the salmon fillets on a baking dish and sprinkle with olive oil liberally. Season with salt and pepper, then sprinkle with lemon zest and thyme equally. Arrange the lemon slices on top of the fillets and top with the garlic cloves.
- Bake for 18-20 minutes, or until the salmon is cooked through and flakes with a fork (modify the baking time if your fillets are very thick or thin).

NOTES:

- This recipe is readily scaled up or down.

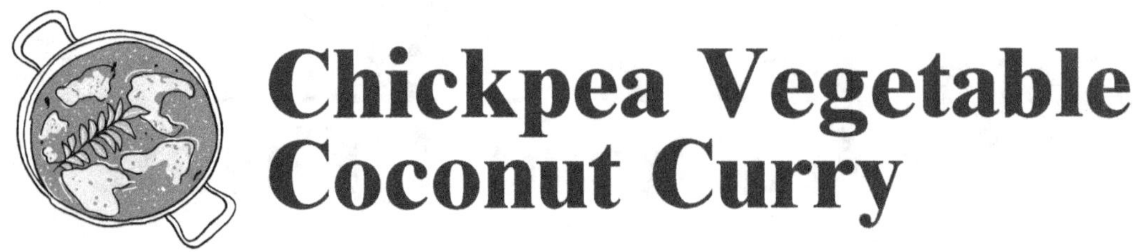

Chickpea Vegetable Coconut Curry

 **PREP TIME:** 10mins	 **COOK TIME:** 10mins	 **SERVINGS:** 4	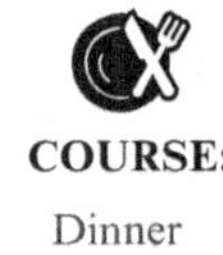 **COURSE:** Dinner

Nutritional Value:	Calories: 665kcal	Fat: 31g	Carb: 80g	Protein: 26g

INGREDIENTS:

- 1 tablespoon extra-virgin olive oil
- 1 red onion, thinly sliced
- 1 red bell pepper, thinly sliced
- 1 tablespoon fresh ginger, minced
- 3 garlic cloves, minced
- 1 small head cauliflower, cut into bite-size florets
- 2 teaspoons chili powder
- 1 teaspoon ground coriander
- 3 tablespoons red curry paste
- One 14-ounce can coconut milk
- 1 lime, halved
- One 28-ounce can chickpeas
- 1½ cups frozen peas
- Kosher salt and freshly ground black pepper
- Steamed rice, for serving (optional)
- ¼ cup chopped fresh cilantro
- 4 scallions, thinly sliced

DIRECTIONS:

- Warm the olive oil in a large saucepan over medium heat. Cook until the onion and bell pepper are nearly cooked, about 5 minutes. Cook until the ginger and garlic are aromatic, about 1 minute.

- Toss in the cauliflower until fully combined. Cook for 1 minute, stirring in the chili powder, coriander, and red curry paste, until the mixture begins to caramelize.

- Stir in the coconut milk and bring to a boil over medium-low heat. Cover the saucepan and continue to cook for 8 to 10 minutes, or until the cauliflower is soft.

- Remove the lid and whisk the lime juice into the curry to mix. Return the mixture to a simmer after adding the chickpeas and peas, seasoning with salt and pepper.

- If preferred, serve with rice. 1 tablespoon cilantro and 1 tablespoon scallions should be garnished on each serving.

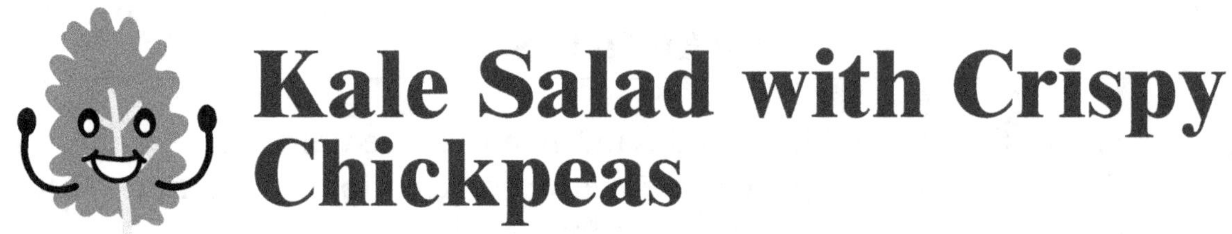

Kale Salad with Crispy Chickpeas

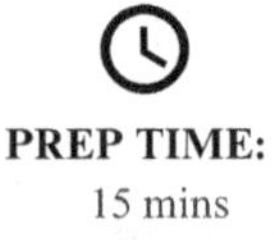 PREP TIME: 15 mins	 COOK TIME: 15 mins	 SERVINGS: 6	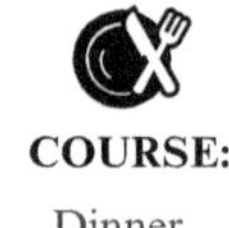 COURSE: Dinner

Crispy Chickpeas	Calories: 229kcal	Fat: 8g	Carb: 31g	Protein: 10g
Dressing	Calories: 170kcal	Fat: 18g	Carb: 1g	Protein: 1g
Kale Salad	Calories: 45kcal	Fat: 2g	Carb: 4g	Protein: 4g

INGREDIENTS:

CRISPY CHICKPEAS

- One 28-ounce can of chickpeas, drained
- 2 tablespoons extra-virgin olive oil
- Zest of 1 lemon
- 1 teaspoon smoked paprika
- Salt and freshly ground black pepper

DRESSING

- 4 anchovies
- 1 garlic clove, smashed
- ½ teaspoon salt
- 1 tablespoon Dijon mustard
- Juice of 1 lemon
- ½ cup extra-virgin olive oil
- ½ teaspoon freshly ground black pepper

KALE SALAD

- 1 large bunch lacinato kale, shredded
- ⅓ cup Parmesan cheese

DIRECTIONS:

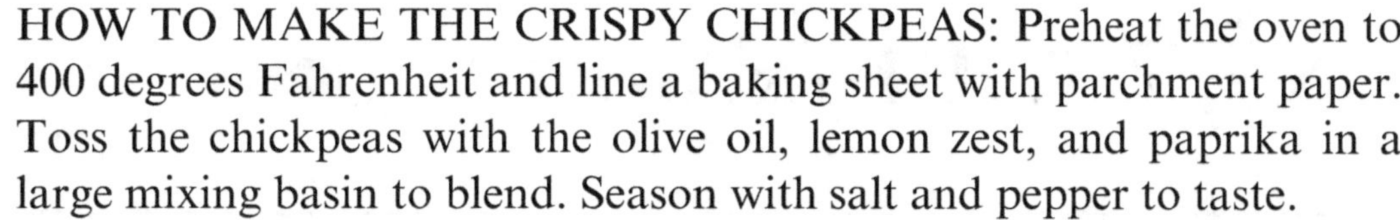

HOW TO MAKE THE CRISPY CHICKPEAS: Preheat the oven to 400 degrees Fahrenheit and line a baking sheet with parchment paper. Toss the chickpeas with the olive oil, lemon zest, and paprika in a large mixing basin to blend. Season with salt and pepper to taste.

Spread the chickpeas in an equal layer on the prepared baking sheet and roast for 40 to 45 minutes, or until very crisp. During cooking, stir the chickpeas once or twice. Allow to cool till room temperature.

MAKE THE DRESSING: Mash the anchovies, garlic, and salt together in a medium bowl. Mix in the mustard and lemon juice thoroughly.

Whisk in the olive oil gently to blend. Season with pepper to taste.

ASSEMBLE THE SALAD: Toss the kale with the dressing in a large mixing bowl. Serve with the cooled chickpeas on top. Using a vegetable peeler, shave the Parmesan into big curls. Serve right away.

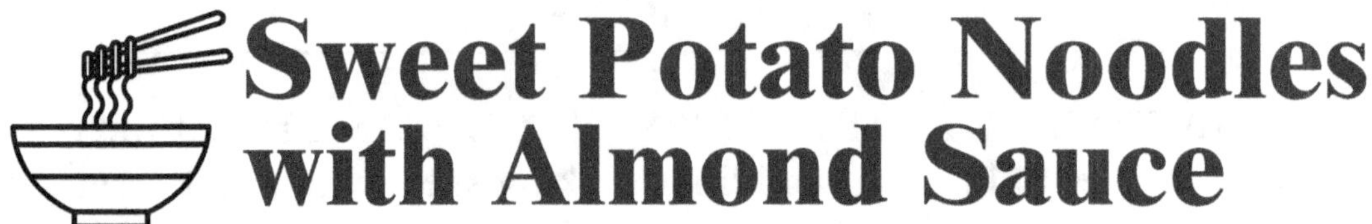

Sweet Potato Noodles with Almond Sauce

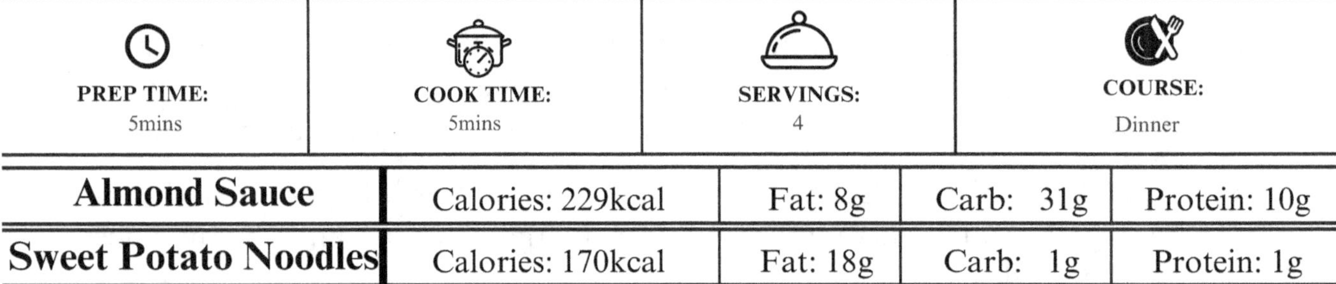

	PREP TIME: 5mins	COOK TIME: 5mins	SERVINGS: 4	COURSE: Dinner
Almond Sauce	Calories: 229kcal	Fat: 8g	Carb: 31g	Protein: 10g
Sweet Potato Noodles	Calories: 170kcal	Fat: 18g	Carb: 1g	Protein: 1g

INGREDIENTS:

ALMOND SAUCE

- 2 tablespoons extra-virgin olive oil

- 3 shallots, minced

- 2 garlic cloves, minced

- 3 tablespoons all-purpose flour

- 2 cups plain, unsweetened almond milk

- 2 tablespoons Dijon mustard

- Salt and freshly ground black pepper

SWEET POTATO NOODLES

- 2 tablespoons extra-virgin olive oil

- 3 sweet potatoes, cut into noodles (made using a spiralizer)

- 4 cups roughly torn kale

- Salt and freshly ground black pepper

- ½ cup toasted, salted almonds, roughly chopped

DIRECTIONS:

- **HOW TO MAKE ALMOND SAUCE:** Warm the olive oil in a medium saucepan over medium heat. Cook until the shallots and garlic are aromatic, about 1 minute.

- Cook, stirring frequently, for 1 minute after adding the flour. Whisk in the almond milk regularly to prevent lumps from forming in the sauce. Whisk the mixture over medium heat until it reaches a simmer. Cook for 4 to 5 minutes.

- Season the sauce with salt and pepper after whisking in the Dijon mustard. While you cook the noodles, cover and keep the sauce heated over low heat.

- **HOW TO MAKE SWEET POTATO NOODLES:** Heat the olive oil in a large sauté pan over medium heat. Cook, stirring periodically, until the sweet potato noodles are nearly cooked, 5 to 6 minutes.

- Toss in the kale until it wilts. Toss in the sauce until the noodles are fully coated.

- Add the almonds and stir to blend just before serving. Season with salt and pepper to taste. Serve right away.

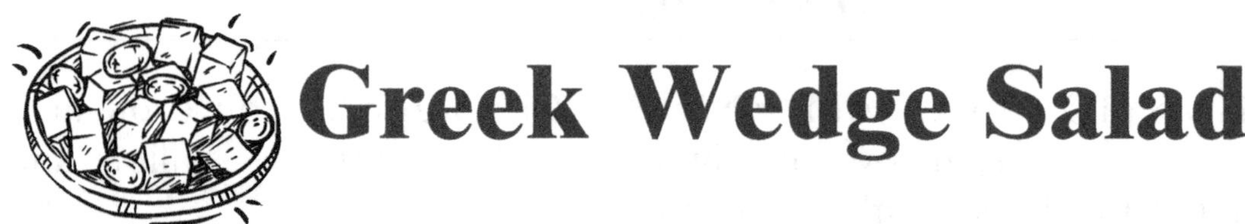

Greek Wedge Salad

   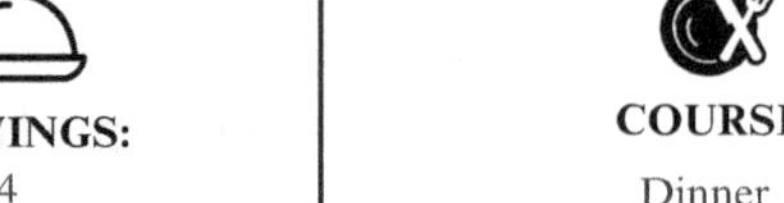

PREP TIME: 15mins	**COOK TIME:** 15mins	**SERVINGS:** 4	**COURSE:** Dinner

Dressing	Calories: 248kcal	Fat: 27g	Carb: 1g	Protein: 0g
Salad	Calories: 153kcal	Fat: 8g	Carb: 18g	Protein: 6g

INGREDIENTS:

DRESSING

- ½ cup extra-virgin olive oil
- 1 tablespoon Dijon mustard
- 1 garlic clove, minced
- 1 teaspoon dried oregano
- 1 teaspoon salt
- ¾ teaspoon freshly ground black pepper
- ⅓ cup red wine vinegar

SALAD

- 1 head iceberg lettuce—washed, cored, and quartered
- 1-pint cherry tomatoes, quartered
- ½ cucumber, thinly sliced
- ½ red onion, thinly sliced
- ½ cup crumbled feta cheese
- 1 cup kalamata olives
- 4 peperoncino peppers

DIRECTIONS:

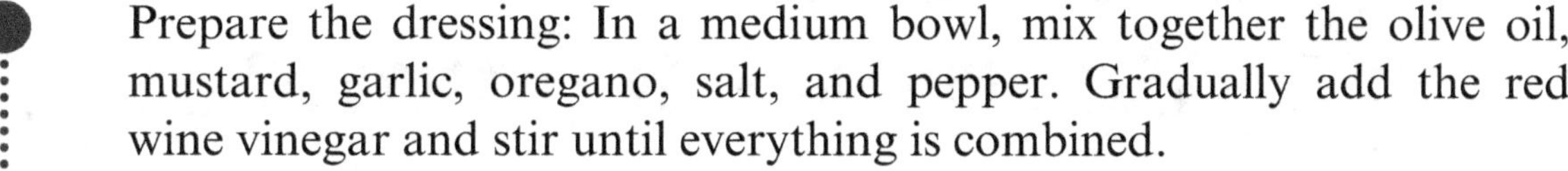

- Prepare the dressing: In a medium bowl, mix together the olive oil, mustard, garlic, oregano, salt, and pepper. Gradually add the red wine vinegar and stir until everything is combined.

- Assemble the salad: Place a quarter of iceberg lettuce on each plate and top with tomatoes, cucumber, and red onion. Drizzle each plate with the dressing to taste.

- Garnish with 2 tablespoons of feta, ¼ cup of olives, and a peperoncino pepper. Serve right away.

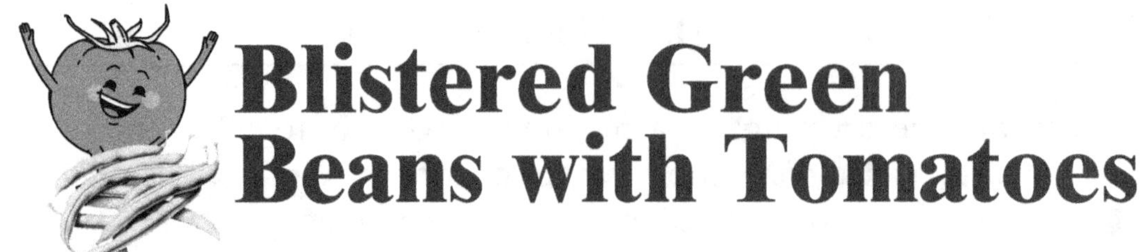

Blistered Green Beans with Tomatoes

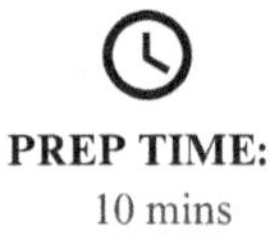			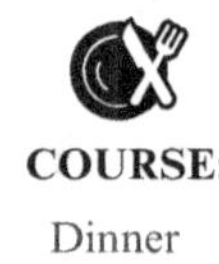
PREP TIME: 10 mins	**COOK TIME:** 10mins	**SERVINGS:** 4	**COURSE:** Dinner

Nutritional Value:	Calories: 261kcal	Fat: 22g	Carb: 16g	Protein: 5g

INGREDIENTS:

- 1 cup walnuts, toasted
- ½ bunch parsley, roughly chopped
- Zest and juice of 1 lemon
- ¼ cup olive oil
- Kosher salt
- 1 tablespoon neutral oil, like canola
- 1 pound green beans, stems snapped off
- 1 pint cherry tomatoes, halved
- 1 medium summer squash, shaved into paper-thin planks or rounds

DIRECTIONS:

- Place the walnuts in a zipper plastic bag and smash with the bottom of a frying pan until the walnuts are broken up into coarse pieces and some oil has been released
- Stir together the walnuts, parsley, lemon zest and juice, olive oil, and a pinch of salt.
- Heat the neutral oil till it is scorching hot, then add the green beans and season with salt. Allow the green beans to blister before tossing to coat, flipping, and blistering the other side.
- Take the pan off the heat and throw in the tomatoes and summer squash. Serve with the walnut mixture on top.

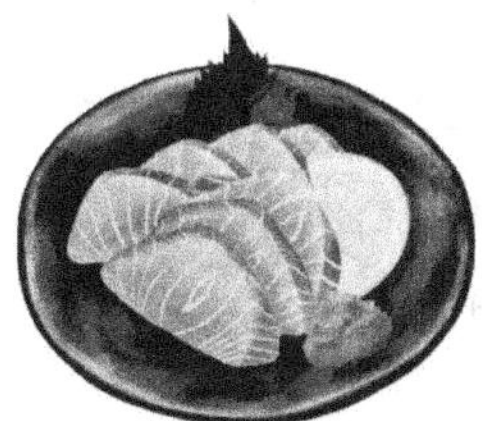

Baked Sesame-Ginger Salmon in Parchment

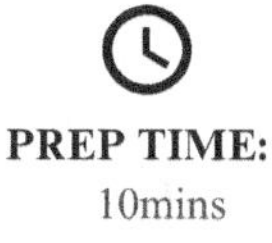 **PREP TIME:** 10mins	 **COOK TIME:** 10mins	 **SERVINGS:** 4	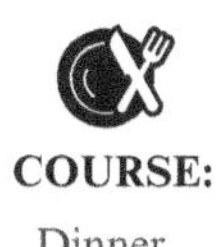 **COURSE:** Dinner

Nutritional Value:	Calories: 468kcal	Fat: 26g	Carb: 21g	Protein: 39g

INGREDIENTS:

- 1 teaspoon sesame oil
- 2 tablespoons soy sauce
- 2 tablespoons grated fresh ginger
- 1 teaspoon garlic powder
- 2 tablespoons honey
- Pinch of red-pepper flakes
- 2 large zucchini, halved lengthwise and thinly sliced
- 1 red onion, halved and thinly sliced
- 1 lime, quartered
- Four 6-ounce skinless salmon fillets
- 4 teaspoons sesame seeds

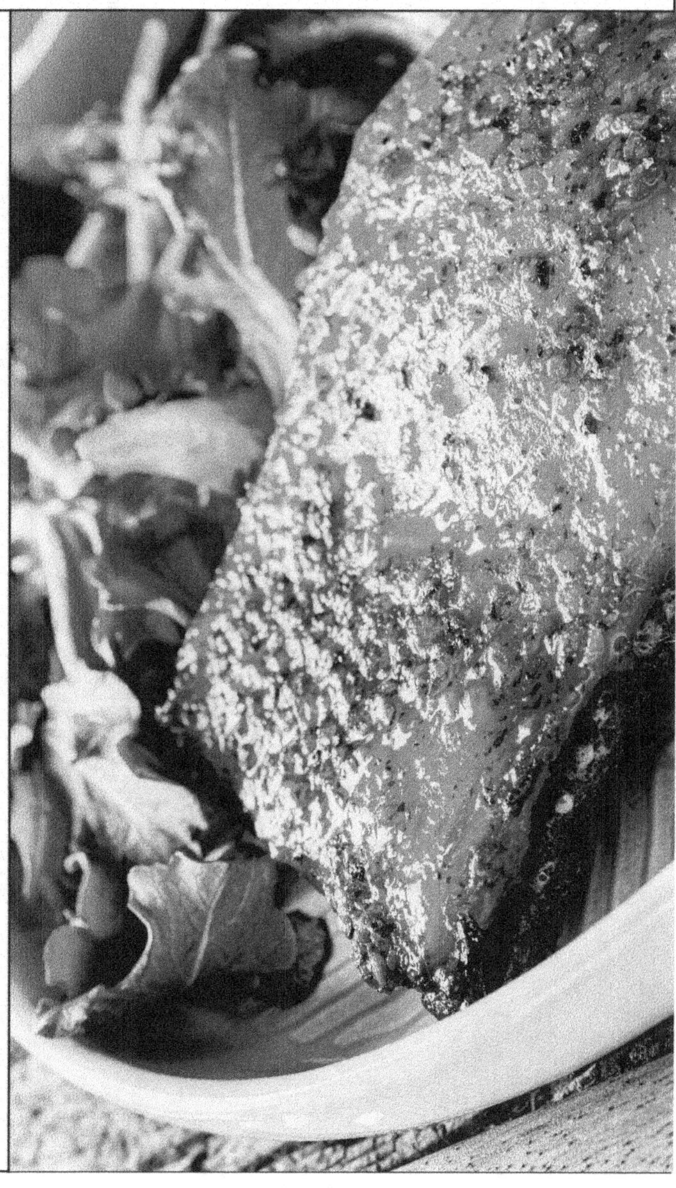

DIRECTIONS:

- Preheat the oven to 350 degrees Fahrenheit. Prepare four 15-by-17-inch pieces of parchment paper. Make a crease in each piece, then unfold and set aside.

- In a small mixing bowl, combine the sesame oil, soy sauce, ginger, garlic powder, honey, and red pepper flakes.

- Make each parchment packet one at a time. Place a quarter of the zucchini in an even layer on one side of a piece of parchment paper, followed by a quarter of the red onion. Squeeze a liberal amount of lime juice over the vegetables.

- Top the vegetables with a salmon fillet. Brush the salmon with the soy sauce mixture and sprinkle with 1 teaspoon sesame seeds.

- To thoroughly seal the package, fold the empty side of the parchment over the salmon and then fold the two sides inward toward the fish, forming multiple creases.

- Rep with the rest of the parchment and materials. Place the prepared packets on a baking sheet and bake for 16 to 18 minutes, or until the salmon is fully cooked.

- Remove the fish and vegetables from the packets and place on plates, or cut slits in the top of the parchment and serve in the paper. Serve right away.

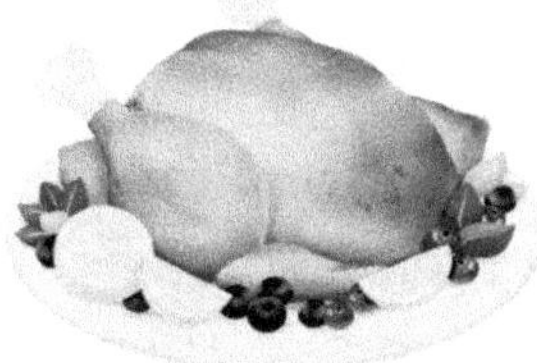

Five-Ingredient Lemon Chicken with Asparagus

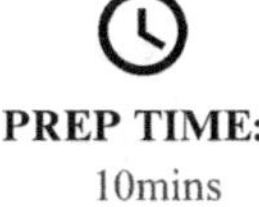 **PREP TIME:** 10mins	 **COOK TIME:** 10mins	 **SERVINGS:** 4	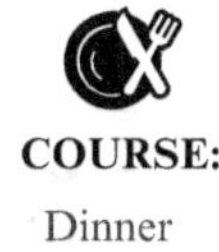 **COURSE:** Dinner

Nutritional Value:	Calories: 232kcal	Fat: 9g	Carb: 1.4g	Protein: 27.5g

INGREDIENTS:

- 1 lb. boneless skinless chicken breasts
- 1/4 cup flour
- 1/2 teaspoon salt and pepper, to taste
- 2 tablespoons butter
- 1 teaspoon lemon pepper seasoning
- 1–2 cups chopped asparagus
- 2 lemons, sliced
- 2 tablespoons honey + 2 tablespoons butter (optional, see FAQ notes)
- parsley for topping (optional)

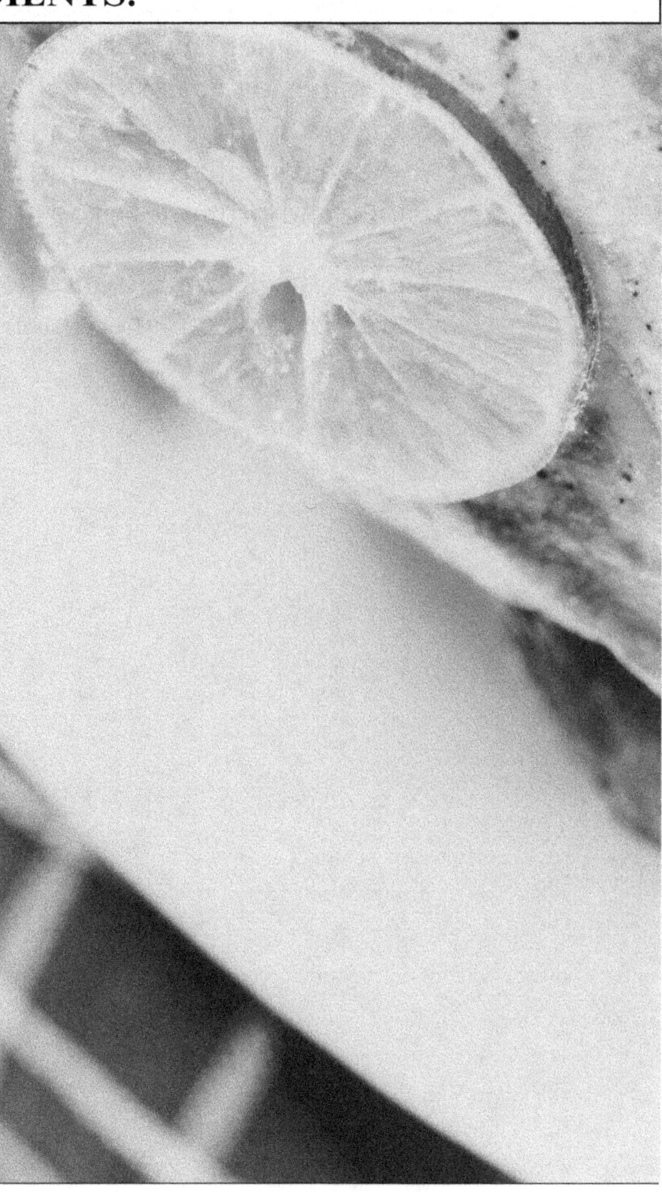

DIRECTIONS:

- Cover the chicken breasts with plastic wrap and use a meat mallet to flatten them to a thickness of 3/4 of an inch. (If the chicken breasts are too thick, you can cut them in half horizontally to make them thinner.)

- Place the flour, salt, and pepper in a shallow dish and lightly coat each chicken breast. Melt the butter in a large skillet over medium-high heat and add the chicken.

- Sauté for 3-5 minutes on each side until golden brown, sprinkling each side with lemon pepper. Transfer the chicken to a plate when it is cooked through. Add the chopped asparagus to the pan and sauté until bright green and tender-crisp.

- Place the lemon slices flat on the bottom of the pan and cook for a few minutes on each side without stirring, so they caramelize and pick up the browned bits left in the pan from the chicken and butter. (Adding a small pat of butter with the lemons also helps prevent sticking and promotes browning.)

- Remove the lemons from the pan and set aside. Finally, layer the asparagus, chicken, and lemon slices back into the skillet.

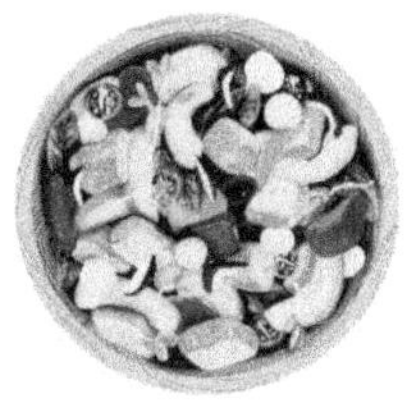

Panzanella Salad

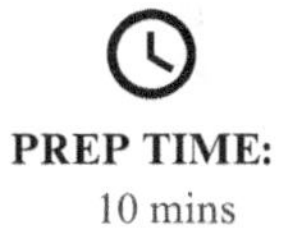	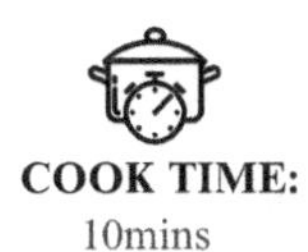		
PREP TIME: 10 mins	**COOK TIME:** 10mins	**SERVINGS:** 1	**COURSE:** Dinner

Nutritional Value:	Calories: 786kcal	Fat: 55g	Carb: 52g	Protein: 24g

INGREDIENTS:

- 2 tablespoons extra-virgin olive oil
- 2½ teaspoons balsamic vinegar
- 1 garlic clove, minced
- ½ teaspoon dried oregano
- Kosher salt
- 1 cucumber, peeled and chopped
- 1 cup cubed stale bread (from a rustic country loaf or baguette)
- 1 cup chopped tomato
- 4 ounces feta cheese, crumbled
- ¼ cup chopped red onion
- 6 Kalamata olives, pitted and chopped

DIRECTIONS:

- Combine the olive oil, vinegar, garlic, oregano, and a pinch of salt in a large mixing basin. Whisk until the mixture is emulsified.

- Combine the cucumber, bread, tomato, feta, onion, and olives in a mixing bowl. Toss the salad with your hands to properly distribute the ingredients. At room temperature, serve.

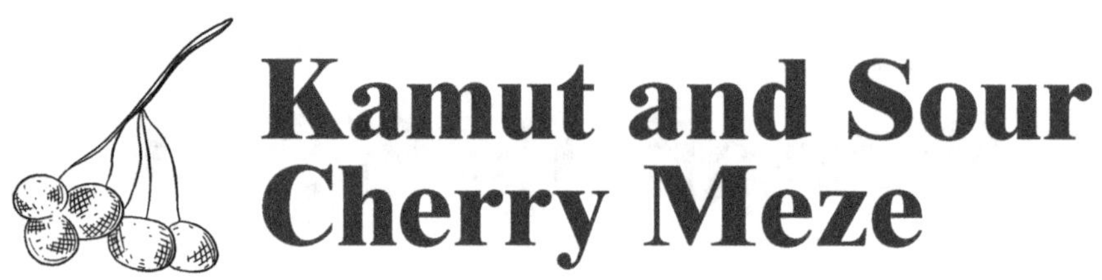 Kamut and Sour Cherry Meze

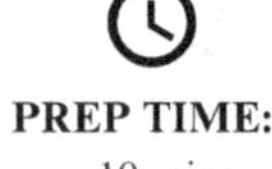 **PREP TIME:** 10 mins	 **COOK TIME:** 10mins	 **SERVINGS:** 6	 **COURSE:** Dinner

Nutritional Value:	Calories: 183kcal	Fat: 8g	Carb: 25g	Protein: 6g

INGREDIENTS:

- 1 cup kamut
- ½ cup chopped dried sour cherries
- ⅓ cup finely chopped toasted walnuts
- ⅓ cup finely chopped fresh parsley
- ¼ cup finely chopped red onion
- ¼ cup finely chopped fresh dill, plus more sprigs for serving
- 2 tablespoons extra-virgin olive oil
- 1 tablespoon lemon juice
- 1 garlic clove, grated
- 1 teaspoon kosher teaspoon salt
- ¼ teaspoon freshly ground black pepper
- ¼ cup feta cheese

DIRECTIONS:

- Bring 3 cups salted water to a boil, then add the Kamut, cover, and lower to a low heat. Cook until the potatoes are soft, about 50 to 60 minutes.

- Toss together the Kamut, cherries, walnuts, parsley, red onion, and dill.

- In a medium mixing bowl, combine the olive oil, lemon juice, garlic, salt, and pepper. Drizzle the dressing over the Kamut and sprinkle with the feta and dill sprigs to decorate.

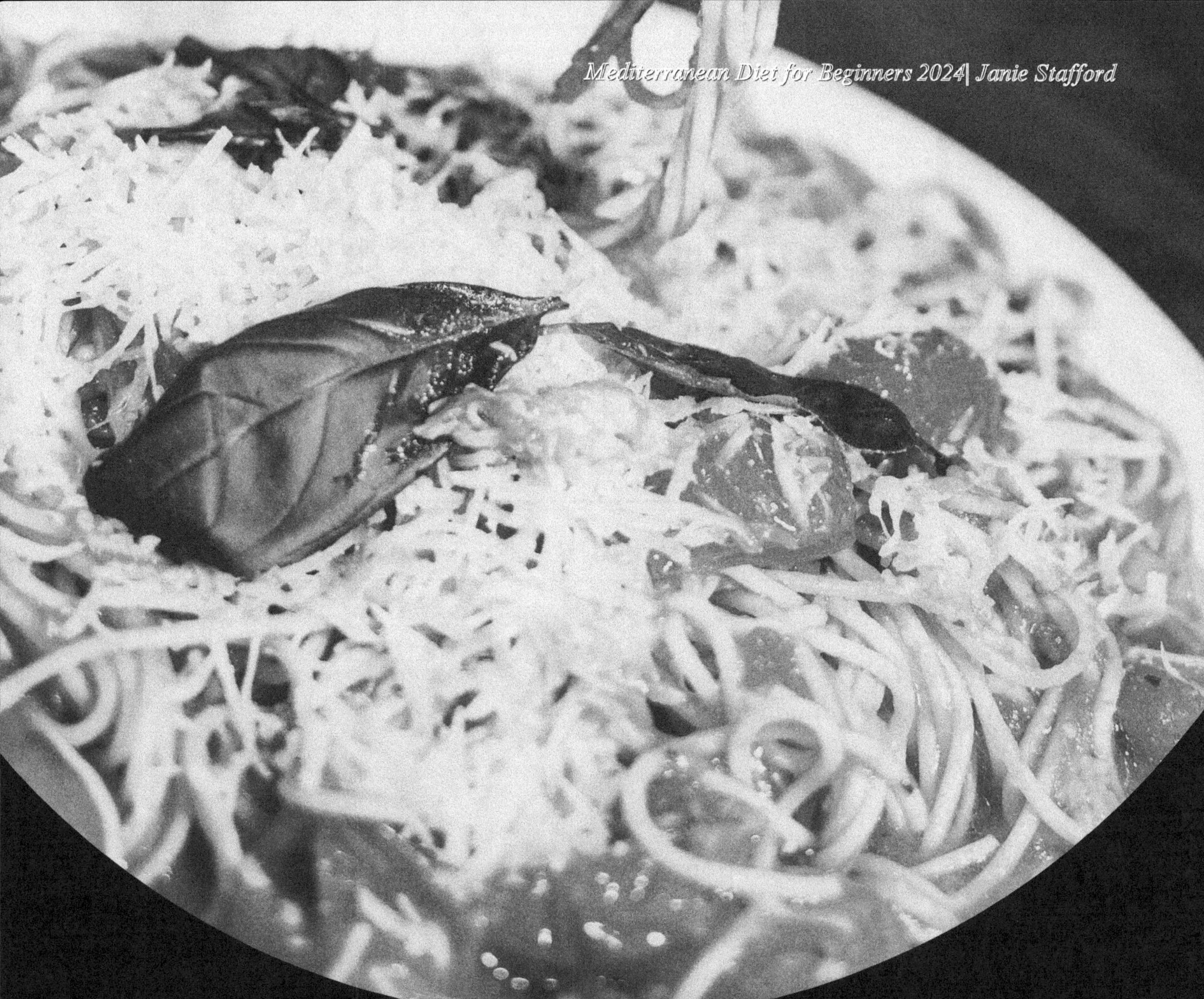

BEANS, GRAINS AND PASTA
RECIPES

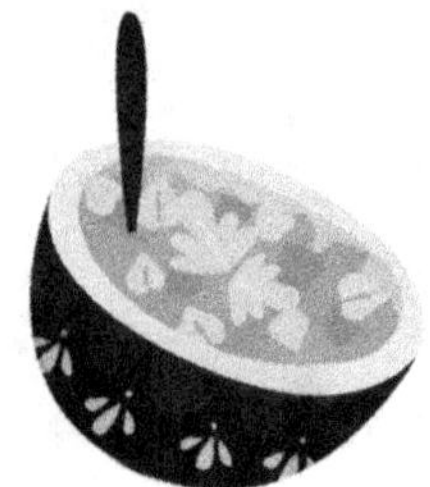

Roasted Cauliflower and Chickpea Stew

			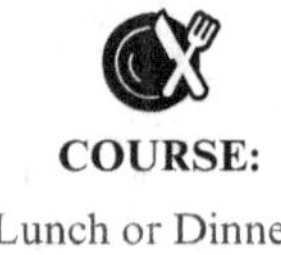
PREP TIME: 10mins	**COOK TIME:** 50mins	**SERVINGS:** Up to 6	**COURSE:** Lunch or Dinner

Nutritional Value:	Calories: 286kcal	Fat: 12.5g	Carb: 37.1g	Protein: 11g

INGREDIENTS:

- 1 ½ tsp ground turmeric
- 1 ½ tsp ground cumin
- 1 ½ tsp ground cinnamon
- 1 tsp ground coriander
- 1 tsp Sweet paprika
- 1 tsp cayenne pepper (optional)
- ½ tsp ground green cardamom
- 1 whole head cauliflower, divided into small florets
- 5 medium-sized bulk carrots, peeled, cut into 1 ½" pieces
- Salt and pepper
- Private Reserve extra virgin olive oil
- 1 large sweet onion, chopped
- 6 garlic cloves, chopped
- 2 14-oz cans chickpeas, drained and rinsed
- 1 28-oz can diced tomatoes with its juice
- ½ cup parsley leaves, stems removed, roughly chopped
- Toasted slivered almonds (optional)
- Toasted pine nuts (optional)

DIRECTIONS:

- Preheat your oven to 475 degrees F. In a small bowl, mix together the spices. Place the cauliflower florets and carrot pieces on a lightly oiled baking sheet. Sprinkle with salt and pepper, then add more than half of the spice mixture.

- Drizzle generously with olive oil and toss to make sure the spices evenly coat the vegetables. Bake for 20 minutes or until the carrots and cauliflower are softened and have some color. Take out of the oven and set aside. Turn off the oven.

- In a large cast iron pot or Dutch oven, heat 2 tablespoons of olive oil. Add the onions and sauté for 3 minutes, then add the garlic and the remaining spices. Cook on medium-high for 2-3 minutes, stirring constantly.

- Add the chickpeas and canned tomatoes. Season with salt and pepper. Stir in the roasted cauliflower and carrots. Bring to a boil, then reduce the heat to medium-low, cover part-way and cook for another 20 minutes. Check the stew, stir occasionally, and add a little water if needed.

- When done, transfer to serving bowls. Garnish with fresh parsley and toasted nuts (optional). Serve hot over some quick-cooked couscous or with a side of warm pita bread. Enjoy!

NOTES:

- How Should You Serve Chickpea Stew? This chickpea stew pairs beautifully with quickcooking couscous or Lebanese rice. Grab a nice pita or some wonderful crusty bread to soak up all the goodness if nothing else.

- Leftovers? This dish serves a small group of 6 people. It will keep nicely in a tight-lid jar and refrigerated for about 4 days. Because there is no cream in this recipe, leftover cooked chickpea stew can be readily frozen. Before storing the stew in freezer-safe containers, make sure it has totally cooled.

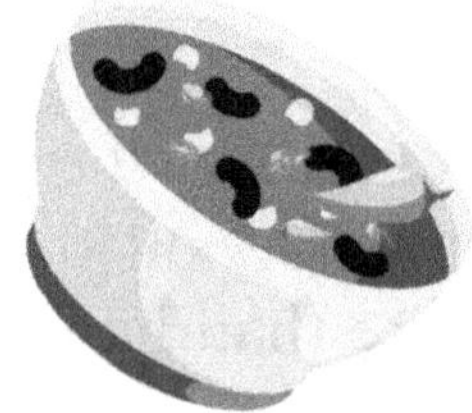

Bean Soup with Tomato Pesto

 **PREP TIME:** 10mins	 **COOK TIME:** 27mins	 **SERVINGS:** Up to 8	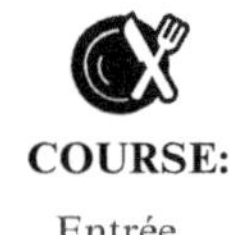 **COURSE:** Entrée

Nutritional Value:	Calories: 366.1kcal	Fat: 20.2g	Carb: 37.3g	Protein: 14g

INGREDIENTS:

- Extra virgin olive oil
- 1 Large russet potato peeled, diced into small cubes
- 1 medium yellow onion chopped
- 1 15- oz can diced tomatoes
- 1 tablespoon white vinegar
- 1 tablespoon ground coriander
- 1 teaspoon Spanish paprika
- Salt and pepper
- 5 cups low sodium vegetable broth, or broth of your choice
- 8- oz frozen spinach, no need to thaw
- 15- oz can red kidney beans, drained and rinsed
- 15- oz can cannellini beans, drained and rinsed
- 15- oz can chickpeas, drained
- Basil leaves for garnish optional
- ⅓ cup toasted pine nuts for garnish optional

For Tomato Pesto Sauce

- 2-3 large garlic cloves, you can start with less garlic if you're not sure
- 1 ½ cup diced fresh tomatoes
- 15-20 large basil leaves
- ½ cup Private Reserve Greek extra virgin olive oil
- Salt and pepper
- ⅓ cup grated Parmesan cheese

DIRECTIONS:

- Heat two tablespoons olive oil in a large Dutch oven or heavy pot over medium heat until shimmering but not smoking. Combine the diced potatoes and onions in a mixing bowl. Cook for 4-5 minutes, tossing frequently.

- Combine the canned diced tomatoes, vinegar, spices, salt, and pepper in a mixing bowl. To blend, stir everything together. Cook for another 4 minutes, covered.

- Remove the cover and add the veggie broth and frozen spinach. Increase the heat to mediumhigh and bring to a boil for about 4 minutes. Combine the kidney beans, cannellini beans, and chickpeas in a mixing bowl. Return to a boil, then lower to a medium-low heat. Cook for another 15 to 20 minutes, covered (potatoes should be soft at this time).

- Make the tomato pesto while the soup is cooking. Place the garlic and fresh tomatoes in the bowl of a food processor fitted with a blade. To blend, pulse a few times. Puree the basil in a food processor. Drizzle in the olive oil a little at a time while the processor is running. In a mixing bowl, combine the thick tomato pesto and the grated Parmesan.

- Remove the soup from the heat when it is done. Incorporate the tomato pesto.

- Serve in serving dishes. Add a few basil leaves and roasted pine nuts to each bowl. With your favorite crusty bread, enjoy!

NOTES:

- If you're looking to make this bean soup for a crowd or to meal prep for several lunches, you can store the leftovers in a glass container with a tight lid and keep it in the fridge for 2-4 days. You can also freeze the cooked soup in portions and thaw it overnight in the fridge before heating it up on the stovetop.

- If you'd like to use dry beans instead of canned, you'll need to start the night before. For each
15-ounce can of beans, you'll need ¾ cups of dry beans. Soak the beans in a large bowl with plenty of water (water to cover the beans by 3 inches) and discard the soaking water before
cooking.

- Put the beans in a cooking pot and cover with water by 2 inches. Bring to a boil, skim off any foam on the surface, reduce heat, cover and simmer gently, stirring occasionally, until the beans are tender, 1 to 1 ½ hours.

- Drain the cooking water and proceed with the recipe as written. You can store the cooked beans in the fridge for 2 days before making the soup, or freeze them for later use.

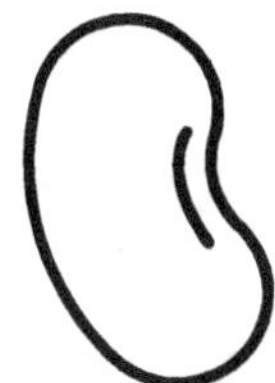

White Bean and Kale Soup with Chicken

			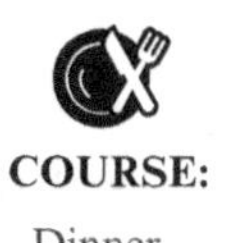
PREP TIME: 10mins	**COOK TIME:** 35mins	**SERVINGS:** 6	**COURSE:** Dinner

Nutritional Value:	Calories: 286kcal	Fat: 1.1g	Carb: 25.1g	Protein: 28g

INGREDIENTS:

- Extra virgin olive oil
- 1 lb boneless chicken cut into small bites
- Kosher salt and black pepper
- 2 medium yellow onions chopped
- 3 garlic cloves minced
- ½ teaspoon red pepper flakes more for later
- ¾ teaspoon ground coriander
- ½ teaspoon ground cumin
- ½ teaspoon dry rosemary
- 2 15- oz cans white beans drained and rinsed, smash contents of 1 can for texture
- 8 cups low-sodium broth chicken or vegetable broth will work here
- 8 oz kale leaves cut into ½ inch strips (no thick stems)
- 2 inch piece Parmesan cheese rind
- 1 to 2 teaspoon fresh lemon juice

DIRECTIONS:

- 2 tablespoon extra virgin olive oil, heated in a big pot. Stir in the chicken. Cook, tossing frequently, until browned (5–7 minutes). Season with kosher salt and freshly ground black pepper to taste. Place the chicken on a separate platter for the time being.

- In the same saucepan, sauté the onions for 4 minutes over medium heat, stirring frequently, until softened (if necessary, add a bit more extra virgin olive oil). Combine the garlic, red pepper flakes, coriander, cumin, and rosemary in a mixing bowl. To blend, stir everything together. Cook, stirring frequently, for 30 seconds to 1 minute over medium heat (be careful not to burn the garlic).

- Return the chicken to the saucepan, along with the white beans (whole and mashed), broth, greens, and cheese rind.

- Raise the heat and bring to a boil for 5 minutes (skim any froth that rises to the surface). Reduce the heat to low. Cover the pot partially, allowing a tiny gap for the soup to breathe. Cook for 25 minutes, or until everything is well cooked and the kale has softened to your preference.

- Take out the cheese rind. Season to taste, adding more of any of the spices used if necessary.

- Finally, add the lemon juice. Serve in serving bowls with a sprinkle of excellent extra virgin olive oil. Serve with crusty bread of your choice.

NOTES:

- Slow Cooker Instructions: Brown the chicken according to package directions (step 1), then transfer to crockpot. Cook on high for 3 to 4 hours or low for 6 to 8 hours with the remaining ingredients EXCEPT the kale. Stir in the greens about 45 minutes before the soup is finished simmering.

- Tip for substituting dry beans for canned beans in this recipe: If you want to use dry white beans instead, you'll need slightly more than 1 cup of dry beans. To begin, soak them in plenty of water overnight.

- Drain and thoroughly rinse with cold water. To prepare the beans for this recipe, place them in a big saucepan and cover with water by 2 to 3 inches. Bring to a boil, scraping any foam that rises to the surface.

- Reduce the heat to low and simmer, partially covered, for 2 hours, or until the beans are tender. Follow the directions above to use cooked beans in this recipe. (If you're cooking white bean soup in the crockpot, soak the dry beans overnight, but you may toss them in the crockpot with the rest of the ingredients and cook until the beans are fully soft.)

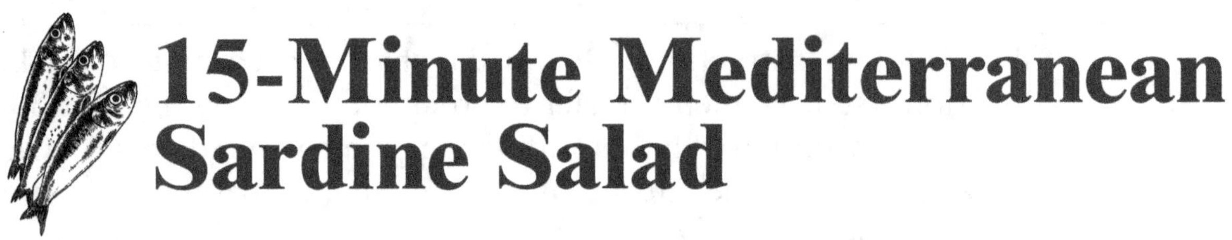 15-Minute Mediterranean Sardine Salad

 **PREP TIME:** 15mins	 **COOK TIME:** 0 mins	 **SERVINGS:** 4	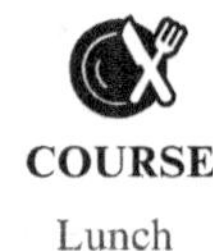 **COURSE:** Lunch

Nutritional Value:	Calories: 239.7kcal	Fat: 7.7g	Carb: 20.9g	Protein: 22.7g

INGREDIENTS:

For The Salad

- 1 can white beans (drained and rinsed)
- 2 cans sardines (4.5 oz cans in olive oil, roughly chopped in large chunks)
- 1 cup cherry tomatoes (halved)
- 2 green onions (chopped)
- 1 to 2 jalapenos (chopped, seeds removed if you don't want the heat)
- 1 cup fresh Italian parsley (chopped)

For The Dressing

- 2 teaspoons Dijon mustard
- 1 lime (zested and juiced)
- 1 to 2 garlic cloves (minced)
- 1 teaspoon sumac
- 1 to 2 teaspoon Aleppo pepper flakes

DIRECTIONS:

- In a small bowl, mix together the mustard, lime zest and juice, garlic, sumac, Aleppo, and a generous pinch of salt and pepper. Whisk the ingredients together and slowly pour in ⅓ cup of extra virgin olive oil while whisking until the dressing is emulsified.

- In a larger bowl, combine the beans, sardines, tomatoes, onions, jalapenos, and parsley. Gently toss the ingredients together.

- Return the chicken to the saucepan, along with the white beans (whole and mashed), broth, greens, and cheese rind.

- Pour the dressing over the salad and mix everything together. Taste and add more seasoning if desired.

NOTES:

- With your favorite crusty bread, this recipe will serve 4 people for lunch. It's more of an appetizer or side dish.

- Use excellent, wild-caught sardines packed in olive oil for the finest flavor. I discussed this further above, but two solutions I've utilized are Wild Planet and King Oscar.

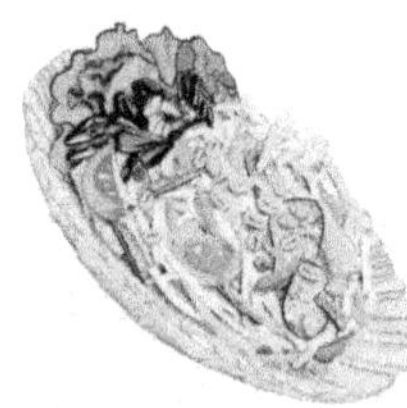

Piyaz: Turkish White Bean Salad

PREP TIME:	COOK TIME:	SERVINGS:	COURSE:
10mins	0 mins	6	Lunch

Nutritional Value:	Calories: 152.6kcal	Fat: 9.1g	Carb: 15.1g	Protein: 4.9g

INGREDIENTS:

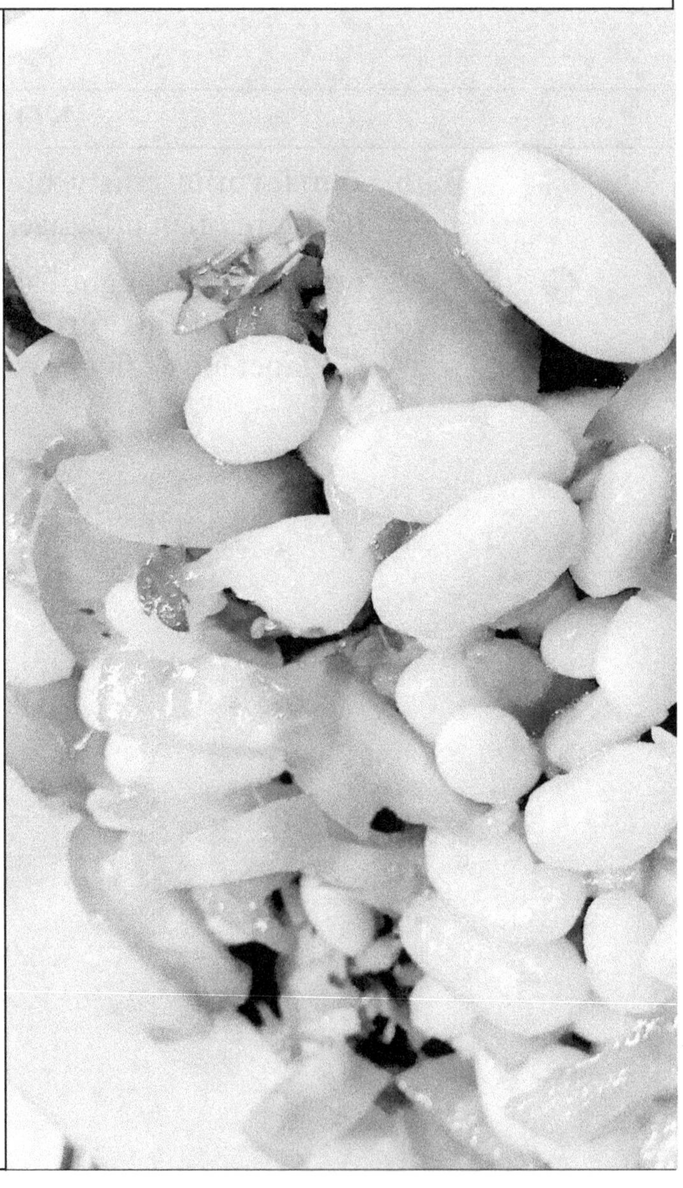

- 1 small red onion, halved and thinly sliced
- 2 garlic cloves, minced
- 5 tablespoons red wine vinegar
- Juice of 1 large lemon
- Kosher salt and black pepper
- 2 teaspoons sumac, more for later
- ¼ cup extra virgin olive oil, our Spanish or Italian EVOO are great options here, given
- their fruity finish
- 1 15- ounce can cannellini beans, drained and rinsed
- 3 Roma tomatoes, cut into wedges
- ½ cup packed chopped fresh parsley

DIRECTIONS:

- Combine the onions, garlic, vinegar, and lemon juice in a large mixing basin. Toss and put aside for about 10 minutes while you work on the rest of the ingredients. (The citrus bath will help to mask the strong onion and garlic flavors).

- Combine the beans, tomato wedges, and parsley in a mixing bowl. Then stir in the sumac, kosher salt, and black pepper to taste. Drizzle the olive oil on top. To mix, toss everything together.

- Season to taste (I frequently add a touch more kosher salt and sumac).

NOTES:

- If you don't have cannellini beans, you can use other white beans such as navy beans, great northern beans, or butter beans. To save time, I used canned beans, but you may instead prepare dried beans from scratch. Just set aside some time for it. You can also substitute another vinegar. Piyaz is typically made using grape vinegar, but white wine vinegar or apple cider vinegar can also be used.

- This Turkish white bean salad goes well with: Piyaz is typically served with Turkish kofte (the dish is known as kofte piyaz). However, for a similar flavor, try it with my shish kofta. It also makes a wonderful fresh side dish alongside chicken doner kebabs and lahmacun. Try it with creamy fried halloumi, eggplant, pink pickles, and your favorite dip on a mezze plate.

- Leftover piyaz will keep in the fridge for about 4 days if stored in an airtight container.

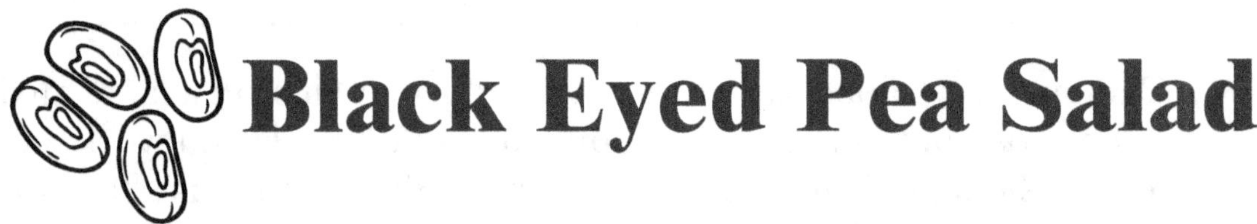

Black Eyed Pea Salad

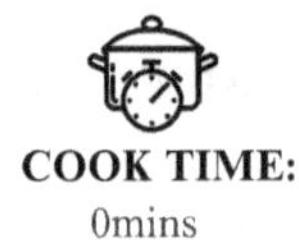 **PREP TIME:** 15mins	 **COOK TIME:** 0mins	**SERVINGS:** 6 people	 **COURSE:** Lunch

Nutritional Value:	Calories: 190.3kcal	Fat: 7.7g	Carb: 25.6g	Protein: 6.5g

INGREDIENTS:

- 15 ounce can black eyed peas, drained and rinsed
- 6 ounces grape tomatoes, chopped
- 1 English cucumber, trimmed and chopped
- ½ cup pomegranate arils, (arils of ½ pomegranate)
- 2 green onions, chopped
- 20 mint leaves, chopped
- Feta cheese, optional

Dressing

- 2 tablespoon pomegranate molasses
- Juice of ½ lemon
- 4 tablespoon extra virgin olive oil
- 1 garlic clove minced
- Kosher salt & black pepper

DIRECTIONS:

- Combine the black eyed peas, diced tomatoes, cucumbers, pomegranate arils, onions, and fresh mint in a large mixing dish.

- Prepare the dressing. Whisk together the pomegranate molasses (or balsamic reduction), lemon juice, olive oil, garlic, and a generous pinch of salt and pepper in a small bowl.

- Dress the black-eyed pea salad with the dressing. To mix, integrate everything thoroughly. Finish with a sprinkling of feta cheese if desired.

NOTES:

- Leftovers: store leftover black eyed pea salad in the fridge in a tight-lid container. If stored properly, it will keep well for 3 days or so.

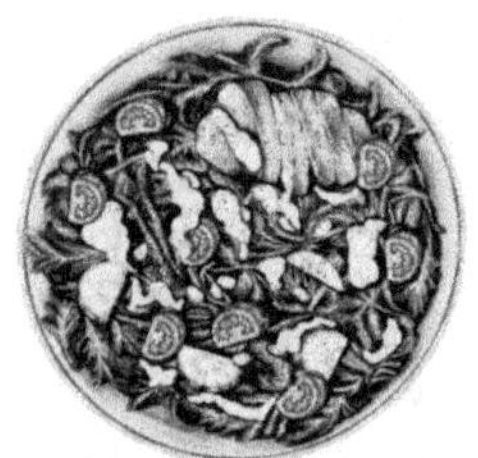

Mediterranean Chickpea Egg Salad

 **PREP TIME:** 15mins	 **COOK TIME:** 0 mins	 **SERVINGS:** 8	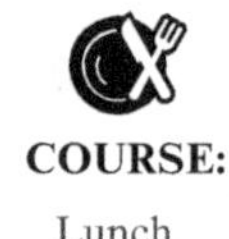 **COURSE:** Lunch

Nutritional Value:	Calories: 193kcal	Fat: 12.9g	Carb: 12.9g	Protein: 7.9g

INGREDIENTS:

For dressing

- 2 ½ tsp Dijon mustard
- 1 large lemon, zested and juiced
- ⅓ cup Private Reserve Greek extra virgin olive oil (or Early Harvest Greek extra virgin
- olive oil)
- 1 garlic clove, minced
- 1 tsp sumac
- ½ tsp coriander
- ½ tsp cayenne pepper
- Salt and pepper

For Egg Salad

- 2 cans chickpeas, rinsed and drained
- 2 celery ribs, chopped
- 2 Persian cucumbers (or ½ seedless English cucumber), diced
- 2 to 3 green onions, trimmed, and chopped (both white and green parts)
- ½ cup shredded red cabbage
- 2 jalapeno peppers, chopped (optional)
- ½ cup packed chopped fresh parsley leaves
- ½ cup packed chopped fresh mint leaves
- 5 large hard boiled eggs, sliced

DIRECTIONS:

- Mix the dressing ingredients in a small bowl or mason jar. Set aside for the time being.

- Combine all of the salad ingredients, except the eggs, in a large mixing bowl. Whisk the dressing briefly before pouring it over the salad. To blend, mix everything together. Mix in the cut eggs carefully one more. Adjust the salt and pepper to taste. Add another sprinkling of sumac. Allow flavors to mingle for a few minutes before serving. (See recipe notes for preparing ahead). Enjoy!

NOTES:

- If you're looking to get a head start, you can mix the salad a few hours before serving

- Make sure to cover it tightly and store it in the fridge. For the best results, add the eggs a few minutes or up to an hour before you're ready to serve.

- The salad will stay fresh for up to three days in a tightly-closed container. If you'd like, you can omit the jalapeno peppers and use mild bell peppers instead. Try using ⅓ to ½ cup of chopped bell peppers of any color you like.

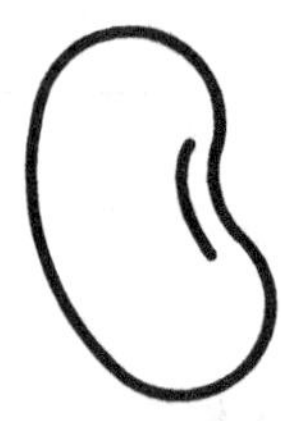

Kidney Bean Salad

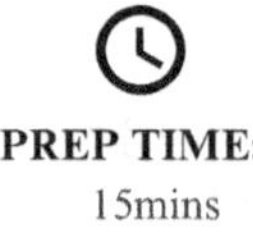 **PREP TIME:** 15mins	 **COOK TIME:** 0 mins	 **SERVINGS:** 4	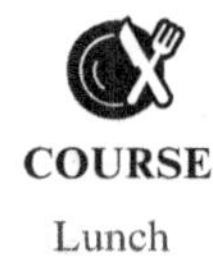 **COURSE:** Lunch

Nutritional Value:	Calories: 154kcal	Fat: 7.4g	Carb: 18.3g	Protein: 5.5g

INGREDIENTS:

- 1 15-oz. can kidney beans, drained and rinsed
- ½ English cucumbers, chopped
- 1 Medium-sized heirloom tomato, chopped
- 1 bunch fresh cilantro, stems removed, chopped (about 1 ¼ cup)
- 1 red onion, chopped (about 1 cup)

Dijon Vinaigrette

- 1 large lime or lemon, juice of
- 3 tbsp Private Reserve or Early Harvest Greek extra virgin olive oil
- 1 tsp Dijon mustard
- ½ tsp fresh garlic paste, or finely chopped garlic
- 1 tsp sumac
- Salt and pepper, to taste

DIRECTIONS:

- Combine the kidney beans, chopped veggies, and cilantro in a medium mixing basin

- To make the vinaigrette, whisk together the lime juice, oil, mustard, fresh garlic, sumac, and pepper in a separate small bowl.

- With a large spoon, blend the vinaigrette with the salad. If necessary, season with salt and pepper

- Refrigerate for 30 minutes to an hour before serving, covered

NOTES:

- Combine the kidney beans, chopped veggies, and cilantro in a medium mixing basin.

- To make the vinaigrette, whisk together the lime juice, oil, mustard, fresh garlic, sumac, and pepper in a separate small bowl.

- With a large spoon, blend the vinaigrette with the salad. If necessary, season with salt and pepper.

- Refrigerate for 30 minutes to an hour before serving, covered.

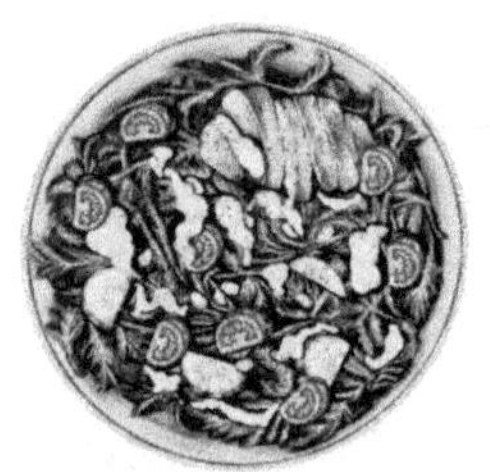

Balela Salad Recipe

PREP TIME:
10mins

COOK TIME:
0 mins

SERVINGS:
6 to 7 servings

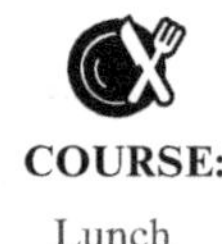
COURSE:
Lunch

Nutritional Value:	Calories: 302.8kcal	Fat: 14g	Carb: 36.8g	Protein: 11g

INGREDIENTS:

For The Salad

- 3 ½ cups cooked chickpeas (or 2 15-ounce cans chickpeas), drained and rinsed
- ½ green bell pepper, chopped
- 1 jalapeno, finely chopped (optional)
- 2 ½ cups grape or cherry tomatoes, halved if you'd like (or you can leave them whole)
- ½ cup sun-dried tomatoes
- 3-5 green onions, chopped (both white and green parts)
- ⅓ cup pitted Kalamata olives
- ¼ cup pitted green olives
- ½ cup chopped parsley leaves
- ½ cup chopped mint or basil leaves

For The Dressing

- ¼ cup extra virgin olive oil
- 2 tablespoons white wine vinegar
- 2 tablespoons lemon juice
- 1 garlic clove, minced
- 1 teaspoon sumac
- ½ teaspoon Aleppo pepper
- ¼ to ½ teaspoon crushed red pepper (optional)
- Kosher salt
- Black pepper

DIRECTIONS:

- Combine the salad ingredients. Combine the chickpeas, bell pepper, jalapeño (if using), tomatoes, green onion, sun-dried tomatoes, olives, and herbs in a large mixing basin.

- Prepare the dressing. Combine the oil, vinegar, lemon juice, garlic, sumac, Aleppo pepper, and red pepper (if using) in a separate bowl or jar. Season with salt and pepper to taste, then mix together.

- Dress. Pour the dressing over the salad and gently toss to coat. Allow for at least 30 minutes before serving, or cover and refrigerate until ready to serve.

- Serve. When ready to serve, give the salad a quick toss and taste to see if the seasoning needs to be adjusted. Enjoy!

NOTES:

- Transform your babela into a meal! This nutritious salad can be quickly turned into a meal. Put it in warm pita pockets with a sprinkle of tahini. Or include it in a vegetarian mezze platter with baba ganoush and roasted red pepper hummus for a delicious spread.

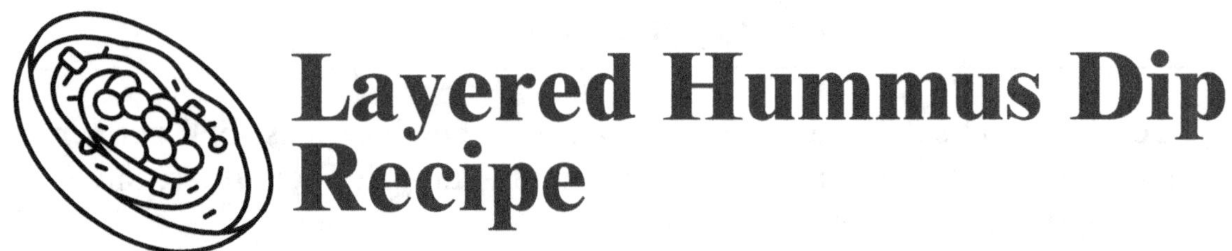

Layered Hummus Dip Recipe

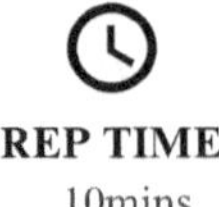	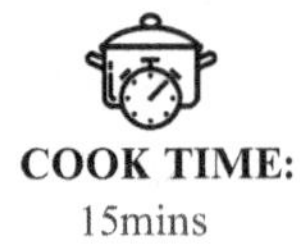		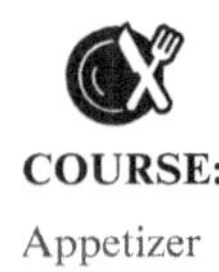
PREP TIME: 10mins	**COOK TIME:** 15mins	**SERVINGS:** 6	**COURSE:** Appetizer

Nutritional Value:	Calories: 246.1kcal	Fat: 14.6g	Carb: 16.1g	Protein: 15.1g

INGREDIENTS:

For Hummus:

- Make this Homemade Hummus Recipe, or use 16-oz store-bought quality hummus that
- you like.
- For Spiced Beef:
- Extra virgin olive oil
- 1 small red onion, chopped, divided
- 2 garlic cloves, minced
- ½ green bell pepper, cored and chopped
- 8 ounces lean ground beef, I used ButcherBox 100% grass-fed and grass-finished beef
- 1 teaspoon ground allspice
- ½ teaspoon sumac
- ¼ teaspoon cinnamon
- ½ cup canned tomato sauce
- Fresh Toppings
- 1 Roma tomato, chopped
- ½ cup chopped fresh parsley
- 3 tablespoon toasted pine nuts, optional

DIRECTIONS:

- To make a delicious layered hummus dip, you can either prepare your own creamy homemade hummus in advance or buy 16-oz of store-bought plain hummus.

- To make the spiced beef topping, heat some extra virgin olive oil in a skillet until it's shimmering.

- Add most of the onions, green peppers, and garlic, and cook over medium-high heat for about 4 minutes until softened. Then add the lean ground beef and sauté until it's fully browned (about 8 minutes).

- Carefully drain any excess fat and season the beef with salt, pepper, allspice, sumac, and cinnamon. Stir in the tomato sauce and cook for another 5 minutes, stirring occasionally.

- To assemble the dip, spread the hummus in a serving bowl and drizzle with quality extra virgin olive oil. Top with the spiced meat, fresh chopped tomatoes, parsley, the remaining red onion, and toasted pine nuts. Serve immediately with warm pita pockets or homemade pita chips. Enjoy!

NOTES:

- Make-ahead advice: If you're preparing hummus from scratch, you may make it a day ahead and refrigerate it. You can also cook the seasoned beef ahead of time.

- What to serve with it: I like to serve it with warm pita pockets or pita chips, but you could also serve it with roasted tomatoes, fried eggplant, or a couscous salad.

- Swaps & substitutions: If chickpeas aren't your thing, try this white bean hummus instead. And don't feel obligated to season the meat in the same way I do! Other warm spices, such as paprika, turmeric, cumin, nutmeg, ras el hanout, and others, can be used.

- Swaps & substitutions: If chickpeas aren't your thing, try this white bean hummus instead. And don't feel obligated to season the meat in the same way I do! Other warm spices, such as paprika, turmeric, cumin, nutmeg, ras el hanout, and others, can be used.

POULTRY AND MEAT

RECIPES

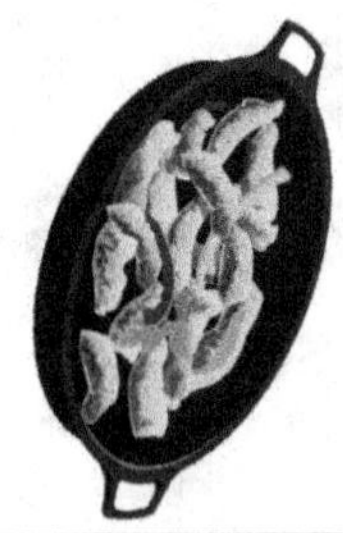

One Pan Chicken and Rice

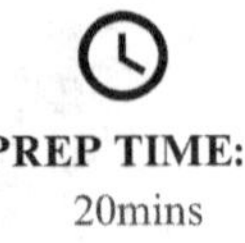			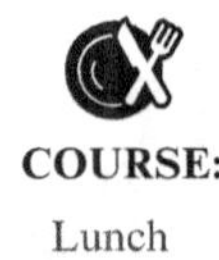
PREP TIME: 20mins	**COOK TIME:** 1hr	**SERVINGS:** 5	**COURSE:** Lunch

Nutritional Value:	Calories: 423kcal	Fat: 29g	Carb: 19g	Protein: 23g

INGREDIENTS:

CHICKEN

- 5 chicken thighs, skin-on and bone-in
- 2 tablespoons olive oil

MARINADE

- 2 lemons, juiced and zested (approx 1/4 cup of juice)
- 2 teaspoons Dijon Mustard
- 3 garlic cloves, minced
- 1 teaspoon dried oregano
- 1 teaspoon dried thyme
- 1/2 tsp salt
- 1/4 tsp black pepper
- 1 tablespoon olive oil

RICE

- 1 yellow onion, diced
- 2 cups baby spinach, lightly packed and roughly chopped
- 2 garlic cloves, minced
- 1 teaspoons dried oregano
- 1 cup long grain white rice
- 2 cups chicken stock
- 1/2 teaspoon salt
- 1/4 teaspoon black pepper
- chopped parsley, for garnish
- lemon zest or slices, for garnish

DIRECTIONS:

MARINATE THE CHICKEN

- In a mixing bowl, combine all of the marinade ingredients.

- Making the marinade for the chicken.

- Place the chicken thighs in a glass dish, pour the marinade over them, and turn to coat. Refrigerate the chicken for at least 30 minutes and up to overnight in a covered dish

- Pour the marinade over the chicken thighs.

COOK THE CHICKEN AND RICE

- Preheat the oven to 350 degrees F. Heat 2 tablespoons olive oil in a large ovenproof skillet over medium-high heat. Cook until the skin on the chicken thighs is golden brown, about 5 minutes. Keep the extra marinade because you'll be adding it back in later.

- In a pan, sear the chicken skin side down.

- Cook for another 5 minutes on the other side. Set aside the chicken thighs from the skillet.

- Scrape and remove any browned bits with tongs, and gather a couple of paper towels to soak up some, but not all, of the fat from the pan. Save some of the fat to sauté the onions in.

- Stir in the diced onions for 1-2 minutes, or until they begin to become translucent.

- In the pan, add the diced onions.

- Combine the chopped spinach, garlic, oregano, salt, pepper, and leftover marinade in a mixing bowl. Stir for 30 seconds more, or until the spinach begins to wilt.

- Stir the rice in the skillet to evenly coat it with the oil.

- Pour in the chicken stock and whisk to combine. On the burner, bring this to a simmer

- Adding the chicken stock and other ingredients to the rice.

- Place the chicken thighs on top of the rice, then cover and bake in the preheated oven. 35 minutes in the oven. Return the skillet to the oven and bake for another 10 minutes, or until the chicken is cooked through and the rice is soft.

- Place the chicken thighs on top of the rice, then cover with the lid

- Allow 5 to 10 minutes for the chicken and rice to rest. As the spinach and onions come to the surface, the rice will appear very black. Before serving, fluff the rice with a fork to bring everything back together.

- Using a fork, fluff the rice in the pan.

- Garnish with chopped parsley and grilled lemon slices or fresh lemon zest if desired.

- The finished chicken and rice recipe with garnishes in one pan.

NOTES:

- To store: Refrigerate any leftover chicken in a sealed container in the refrigerator for 3-4 days.

- To freeze leftovers, place them in a freezer-safe container and place them in the freezer for up to 2 months.

- Reheat the chicken in the microwave for 2 to 3 minutes. Run the chicken under the broiler for a few minutes to crisp up the skin. Just keep an eye on it to make sure it doesn't burn.

- This Staub braiser pan is one of my favorite oven-safe pans. It's quite versatile and well worth the cost!

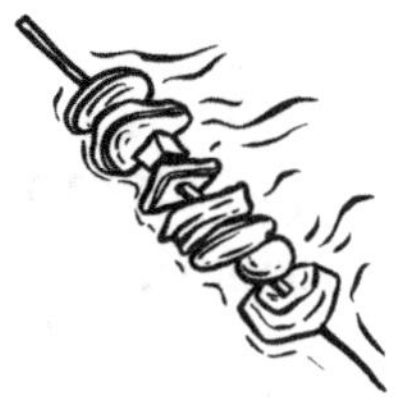

Greek Chicken Kabobs

PREP TIME: 30mins	**COOK TIME:** 25mins	**SERVINGS:** 6 servings	**COURSE:** Lunch

Nutritional Value:	Calories: 135kcal	Fat: 6g	Carb: 11g	Protein: 10g

INGREDIENTS:

MARINADE

- ¼ cup olive oil
- 2 tablespoons red wine vinegar
- 3 tablespoons lemon juice
- 1 teaspoon Dijon mustard
- 3 garlic cloves, minced
- 1 teaspoon dried oregano
- ½ teaspoon salt
- ¼ teaspoon black pepper

CHICKEN KABOBS

- 1 ½ pounds boneless skinless chicken breasts, about 3 large chicken breasts, cut into 1 ½-
- inch pieces.
- 1 red bell pepper, seeded, cut into 1 ½-Inch pieces
- 1 yellow bell pepper, seeded, cut into 1 ½-inch pieces
- 1 red onion, cut into 1 ½-inch chunks
- 1 zucchini, sliced

DIRECTIONS:

- Prepare the marinade. Combine the olive oil, red wine vinegar, lemon juice, Dijon mustard, minced garlic, dried oregano, salt, and pepper in a mixing bowl.

- Making the marinade for the chicken kabobs

- Prepare the chicken by marinating it. Place the chicken in a glass dish and pour the marinade over it. Refrigerate for at least one hour after covering.

- a serving of marinated chicken

- Skewers should be threaded. Preheat a gas or charcoal grill to medium-high. Thread the skewers with red onion, chicken, zucchini, and bell pepper slices. You can change the order.

- Threading skewers with chicken kabobs

- Skewers should be grilled. Cook the kabobs for 4 to 5 minutes per side on a hot grill. After about 15 minutes, the kabobs are done when the chicken is cooked through and the vegetables are lightly browned.

- A grill with skewers of chicken kabob

- Serve with lemon wedges and tzatziki sauce on the side.

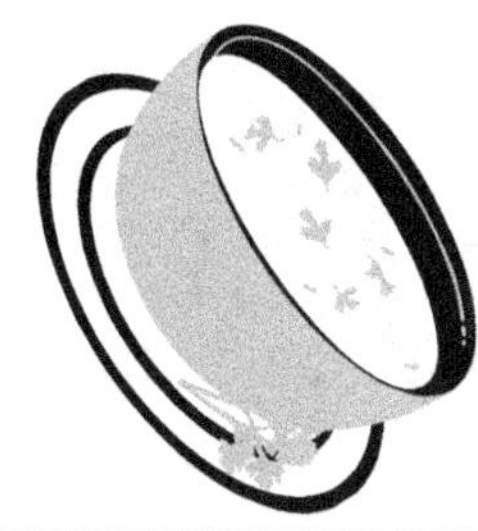

Greek Avgolemono Soup

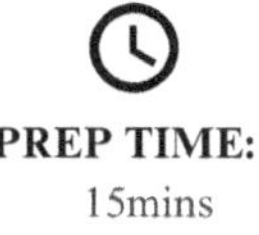 **PREP TIME:** 15mins	 **COOK TIME:** 15mins	 **SERVINGS:** 4	 **COURSE:** Lunch

Nutritional Value:	Calories: 309kcal	Fat: 6g	Carb: 23g	Protein: 27.3g

INGREDIENTS:

- 1 tablespoon extra-virgin olive oil
- 1 small onion, diced
- 2 celery rib, chopped
- 4 cups low-sodium chicken broth
- kosher salt and freshly ground black pepper, to taste
- 2 large eggs
- ¼ cup freshly squeezed lemon juice (from about 1 to 2 lemons)
- 1 ½ cup cooked white rice
- 2 cups shredded chicken
- chopped fresh dill for garnish

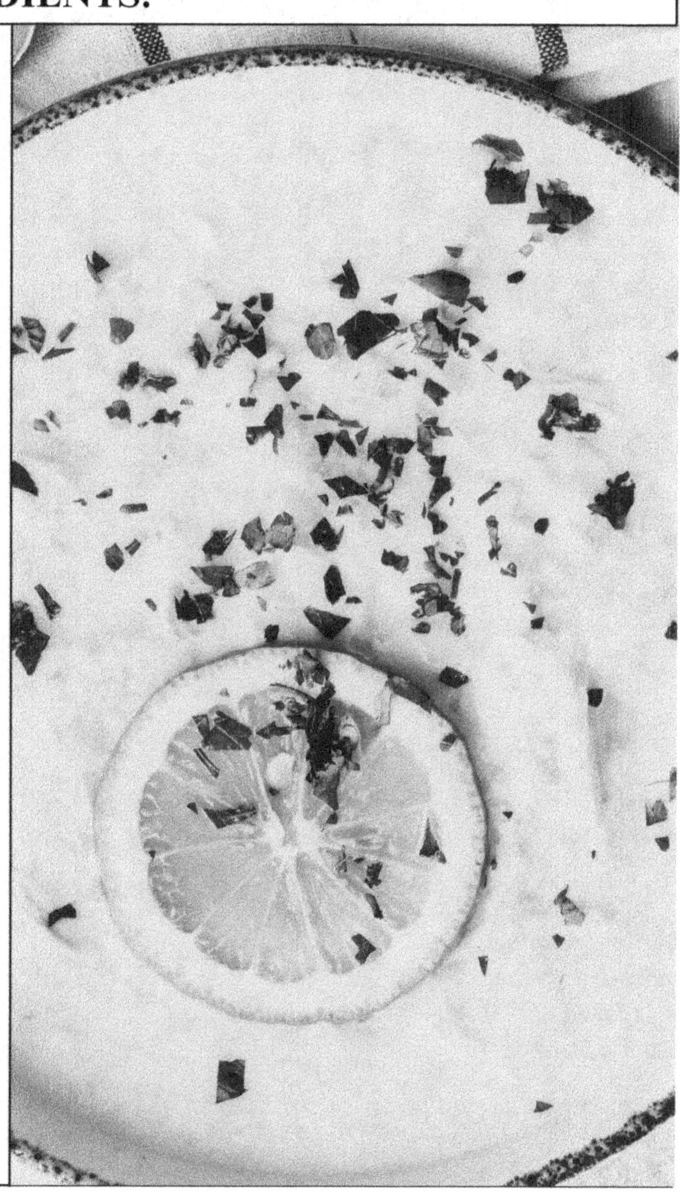

DIRECTIONS:

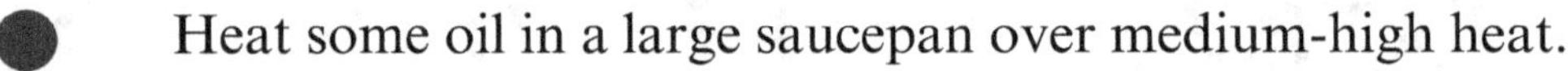

- Heat some oil in a large saucepan over medium-high heat.

- Throw in the onion and celery and sauté for 3 to 4 minutes, until softened.

- Pour in the broth, season with salt and pepper, and bring to a simmer.

- In a blender, add the eggs, lemon juice, and ¼ cup of the rice.

- Blend until smooth, about 20 seconds. Then while blending, slowly stream 2 ladles full of hot broth from the saucepan to temper the eggs.

- Stir the lemon egg puree into the lightly simmering stock along with the rice and chicken, until slightly thickened, about 5 to 10 minutes.

- Make sure not to boil the soup as it can cause the egg mixture to curdle. Finally, garnish with dill before serving.

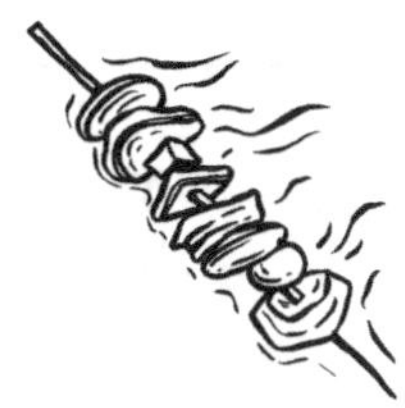

Grilled Chicken Souvlaki

PREP TIME:
30mins

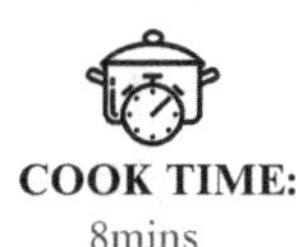

COOK TIME:
8mins

SERVINGS:
4

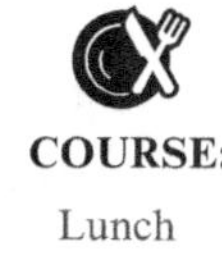

COURSE:
Lunch

Nutritional Value:	Calories: 447kcal	Fat: 34g	Carb: 9g	Protein: 28g

INGREDIENTS:

CHICKEN SOUVLAKI

- 4 boneless skinless chicken breasts, cut into 1 ½-inch cubes
- ⅓ cup olive oil
- 2 tablespoons lemon juice
- 3 cloves garlic, minced
- 2 teaspoons dried oregano
- 1 teaspoon dried parsley
- 1 teaspoon kosher salt
- ½ teaspoon freshly ground black pepper
- 1 recipe tzatziki sauce

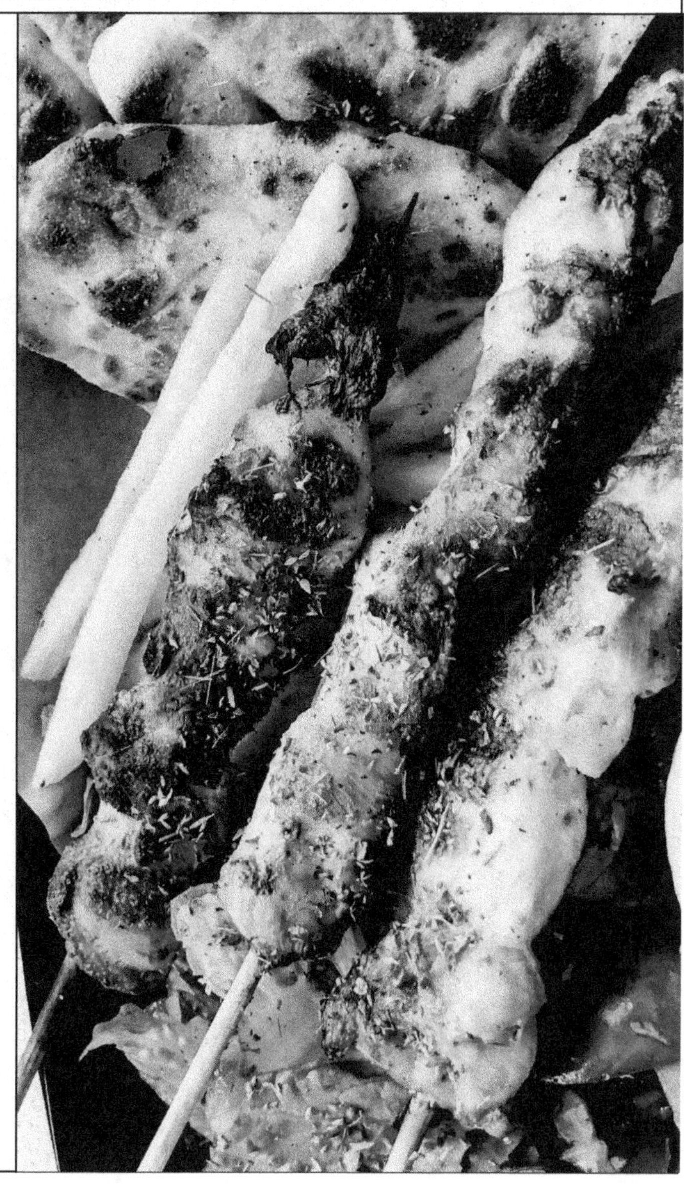

DIRECTIONS:

- In a large mixing bowl, combine the chicken, oil, lemon juice, garlic, oregano, parsley, salt, and pepper. Mix everything together. Place the bowl in the refrigerator for at least 30 minutes to marinate.

- In a glass bowl, marinate the chicken souvlaki.

- Preheat the grill to medium-high. Thread the marinated chicken pieces onto skewers (8 to 9 pieces per skewer = 6 skewers).

- Skewers with chicken souvlaki

- Grill the skewers for 3 to 4 minutes on each side.

- Souvlaki with grilled chicken

- The grilled chicken souvlaki was served with tzatziki sauce.

- A platter of chicken souvlaki with vegetables

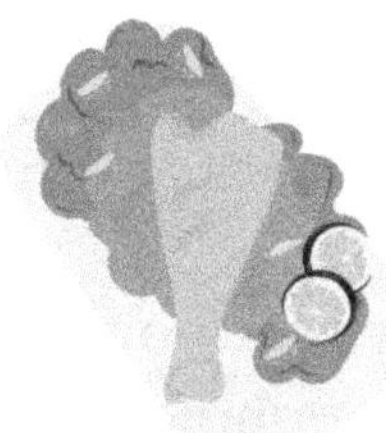

Ultimate Chicken Salad

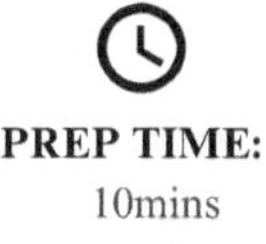 **PREP TIME:** 10mins	 **COOK TIME:** 15mins	 **SERVINGS:** 6	 **COURSE:** Lunch

Nutritional Value:	Calories: 524kcal	Fat: 6g	Carb: 10g	Protein: 36g

INGREDIENTS:

- 2 pounds boneless skinless chicken breasts
- ½ cup sliced raw almonds
- 1 cup mayonnaise
- 1 tablespoon Dijon mustard
- 1 cup red grapes, quartered
- 2 celery ribs, diced
- 3 green onions (green and white parts), sliced
- 2 tablespoon finely chopped parsley
- 1 tablespoon finely chopped tarragon
- 1 lemon , juiced (about 3 tablespoons)
- kosher salt and freshly ground black pepper, to taste

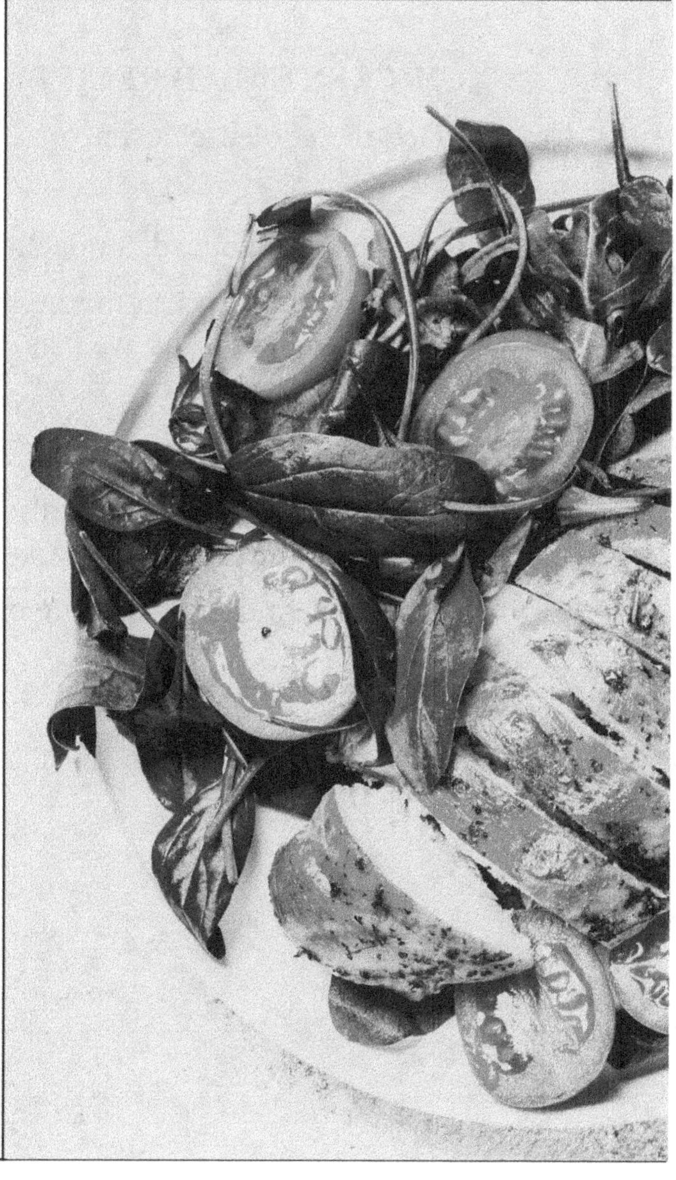

DIRECTIONS:

TO POACH THE CHICKEN

Place two chicken breasts in a pot and cover with cold water, about an inch deep. Add salt to the water and any aromatics of your choice.

Turn the heat to medium until it reaches a gentle simmer, then reduce the heat to low and cover the pan.

Let the chicken simmer for 8 to 12 minutes, or until the internal temperature reaches 160°F to 165°F.

Once done, remove the chicken and let it rest for a few minutes before chilling in the fridge. Follow my poached chicken recipe for more details.

CHICKEN SALAD RECIPE

Place the cooled chicken on a cutting board and cut it into 12-inch pieces.

On a chopping board, a poached chicken.

Chop the celery, green onion, grapes, parsley, and tarragon. Combine those ingredients, as well as the mayonnaise, Dijon mustard, and lemon juice, in a mixing bowl. Season with salt and pepper to taste.

In a bowl, combine the ingredients for the chicken salad.

Combine everything until it's well blended. Allow it to chill in the refrigerator until ready to serve.

Salad with chicken in a white bowl

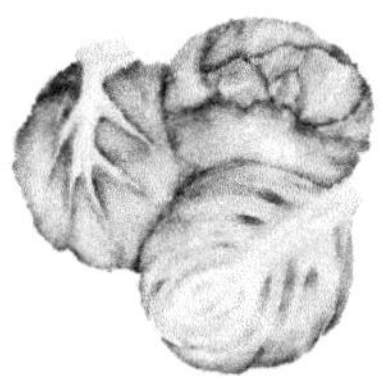

Roasted Balsamic Chicken With Brussels Sprouts

 **PREP TIME:** 2hrs	 **COOK TIME:** 30mins	 **SERVINGS:** 6 servings	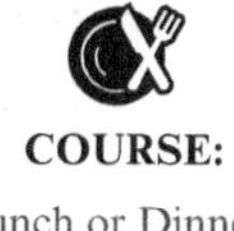 **COURSE:** Lunch or Dinner

Nutritional Value:	Calories: 478kcal	Fat: 34g	Carb: 17g	Protein: 26g

INGREDIENTS:

- ½ cup balsamic vinegar
- 4 tablespoons extra-virgin olive oil
- 2 tablespoons maple syrup
- 3 garlic cloves, minced
- ½ teaspoon kosher salt, or more to taste
- ¼ teaspoon freshly ground black pepper, or more to taste
- 6 chicken thighs
- 1 pound Brussels sprouts, ends trimmed off and sliced in half
- 1 red onion, sliced into wedges

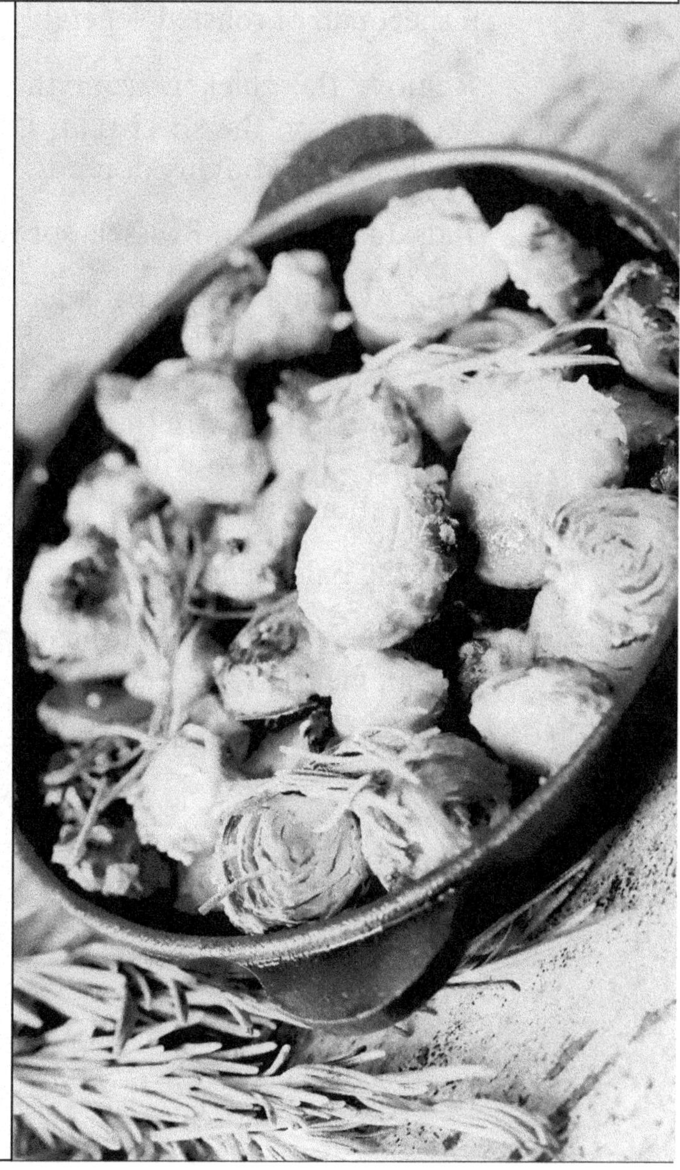

DIRECTIONS:

- Whisk together the balsamic vinegar, 2 tablespoons olive oil, maple syrup, garlic, salt, and pepper in a medium mixing bowl.

- Marinade for balsamic chicken in a bowl

- Pour the marinade over the chicken thighs in a big glass bowl or plastic bag. Marinate for 1 to 2 hours in the refrigerator.

- Chicken thighs marinated in balsamic vinegar

- Preheat the oven to 425 degrees Fahrenheit (220 degrees Celsius). On a sheet pan, arrange the Brussels sprouts and onion. Season with salt and pepper and drizzle with the remaining 2 tablespoons olive oil. Mix everything together on the sheet pan using your hands.

- a sheet pan of roasted vegetables

- Remove the chicken from the marinade and nestle it between the vegetables on the sheet pan. Bake for 30 to 40 minutes, or until the chicken is thoroughly done.

- Balsamic chicken, Brussels sprouts, and onions on a sheet pan

- Pour the remaining marinade into a small saucepan over medium-low heat while the chicken bakes. Simmer for 8 to 10 minutes, or until the sauce has thickened and decreased. Continue roasting the chicken after brushing it with the glaze. Repeat once more while the chicken is baking. The glaze will continue to thicken as it cools, so the second application will be much thicker.

- Making balsamic chicken on a sheet pan

- Serve the chicken after it has reached 165°F (74°C) on an instant read thermometer.

- Dinner on a sheet pan with balsamic chicken and Brussels sprouts

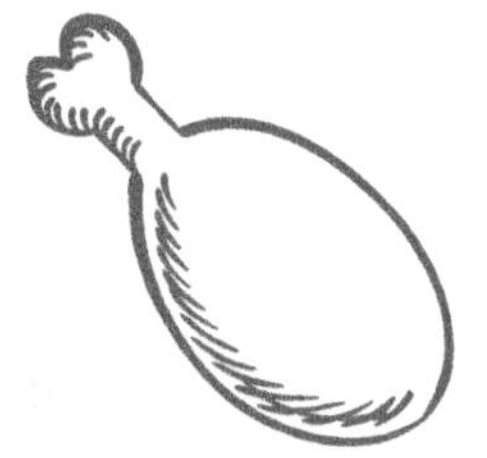

Chicken Soup

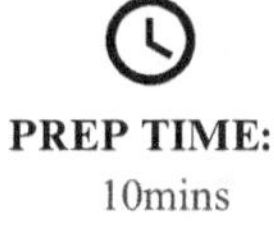			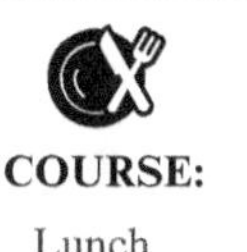
PREP TIME: 10mins	**COOK TIME:** 20mins	**SERVINGS:** 4 servings	**COURSE:** Lunch

Nutritional Value:	Calories: 319kcal	Fat: 2g	Carb: 38g	Protein: 21g

INGREDIENTS:

- 2 tablespoons extra virgin olive oil
- 4 medium carrots, peeled and sliced
- 3 parsnips, peeled and sliced
- 3 celery ribs, sliced
- ½ medium onion, diced
- 1 leek, halved lengthwise, sliced, and rinsed
- 4 garlic cloves, minced
- 1 teaspoon kosher salt
- ½ teaspoon freshly ground black pepper
- 2 boneless skinless chicken breasts
- 2 sprigs fresh thyme
- 2 sprigs fresh tarragon
- 1 bay leaf
- 5 cups low-sodium chicken broth
- ¼ cup roughly chopped fresh parsley

DIRECTIONS:

- Saute the veggies. Heat some oil in a large pot over medium heat. Throw in the carrots, parsnips, celery, leek, and onion and cook for 4 to 5 minutes, stirring regularly. Add the garlic, salt, and pepper, and stir for another minute.

- To make chicken soup, poach the chicken. Put the thyme, tarragon, bay leaf, chicken, and broth in the pot.

- Bring it to a boil, then reduce the heat to low and cover the pot. Simmer the soup for 15 minutes, or until the chicken is cooked through.

- Once the chicken is done, shred it. Take the chicken out of the pot with tongs and shred it with two forks. Put the shredded chicken back into the pot and simmer for an additional 1 to 2 minutes.

- Finally, serve the soup. Remove the sprigs of thyme, tarragon and the bay leaf. Stir in the parsley, and garnish with extra fresh parsley and black pepper before serving.

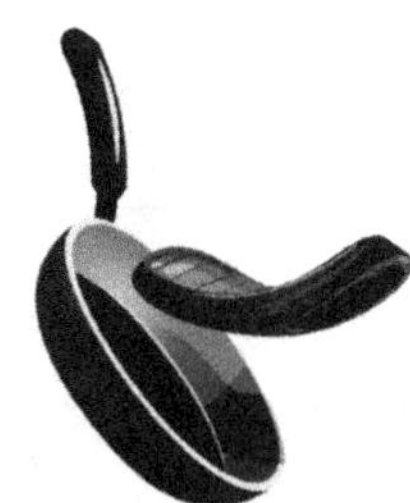

Mediterranean Ground Beef Stir Fry

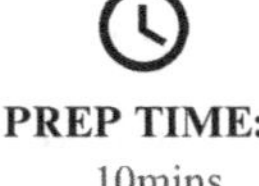

PREP TIME:
10mins

COOK TIME:
15mins

SERVINGS:
4 servings

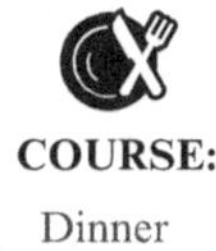

COURSE:
Dinner

Nutritional Value:	Calories: 304kcal	Fat: 17g	Carb: 11g	Protein: 27g

INGREDIENTS:

- 1 tablespoon olive oil
- 1 red bell pepper, deseeded and diced
- 1-pint cherry tomatoes, sliced in half
- 8 ounces baby spinach (small tub)
- 4 garlic cloves, minced
- 2 green onion, thinly sliced, white and green parts separated
- 1 pound ground beef
- ½ teaspoon dried oregano
- kosher salt and freshly ground black pepper, to taste
- 2 tablespoons crumbled feta

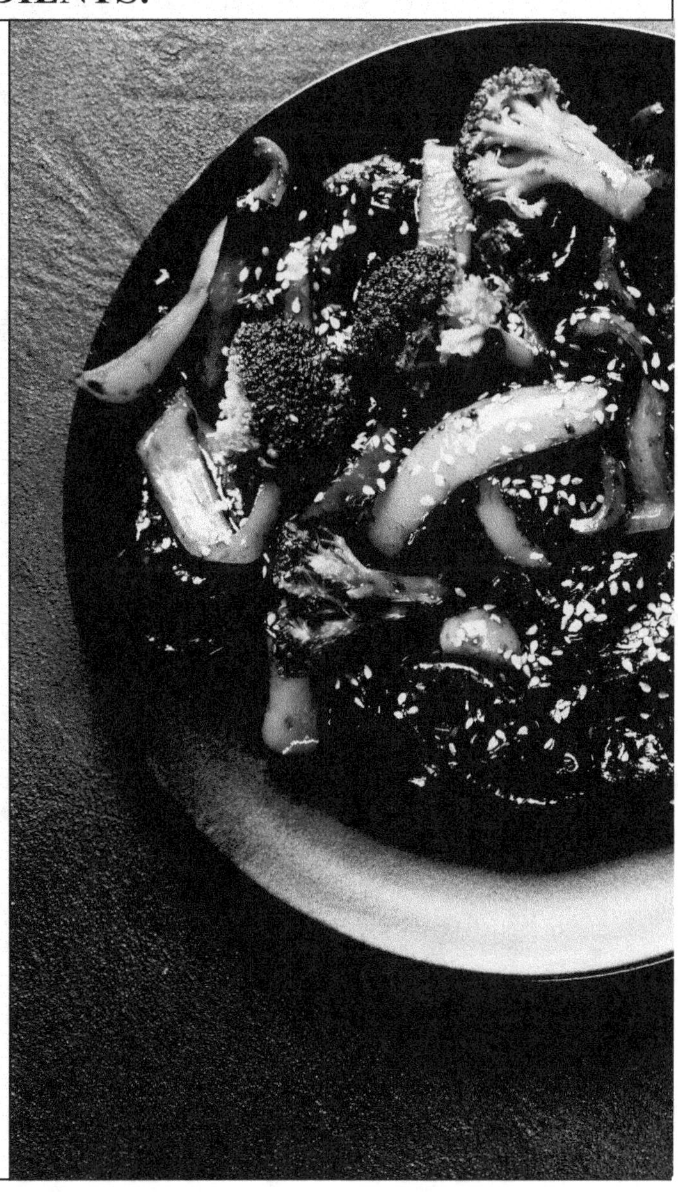

DIRECTIONS:

- In a large skillet over medium-high heat, heat the oil. Cook for 4-5 minutes, or until the bell pepper and cherry tomatoes are blistered and juicy. Stir in the garlic for another minute.

- Mix in the spinach and green onion whites. The spinach will take up the majority of the pan, but it will wilt. Continue to stir for another 2-3 minutes, or until the spinach has wilted. Place these vegetables on a platter.

- Tomatoes and spinach are being sautéed for a Mediterranean ground beef stir fry.

- Add the ground beef, oregano, salt, and pepper to the pan and break it up with a spatula. Cook until the ground beef is browned, then drain any extra fat.

- In a pan, brown ground beef for a stir fry.

- Return the vegetables to the pan and mix in the green sections of the green onion until warmed through. Before serving, top with crumbled feta.

- Stir cook Mediterranean ground beef in a metal pan next to a napkin.

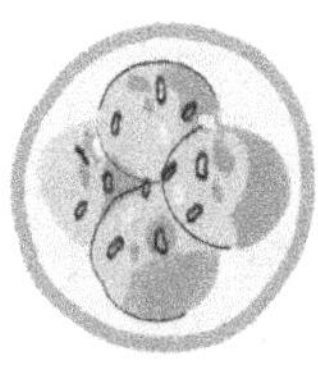

Pork and Fennel Meatballs

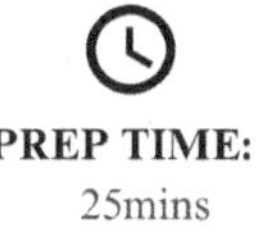			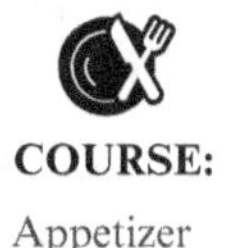
PREP TIME: 25mins	**COOK TIME:** 35mins	**SERVINGS:** 10 servings	**COURSE:** Appetizer

Nutritional Value:	Calories: 308kcal	Fat: 13g	Carb: 2g	Protein: 17g

INGREDIENTS:

- 4 tablespoons olive oil
- ½ medium onion, finely chopped
- ½ fennel bulb, finely chopped
- 2 pounds ground pork
- 2 large eggs, lightly beaten
- ¼ cup roughly chopped fresh parsley
- 1 teaspoon ground fennel seed
- 1 teaspoon kosher salt
- ½ teaspoon freshly ground black pepper, to taste

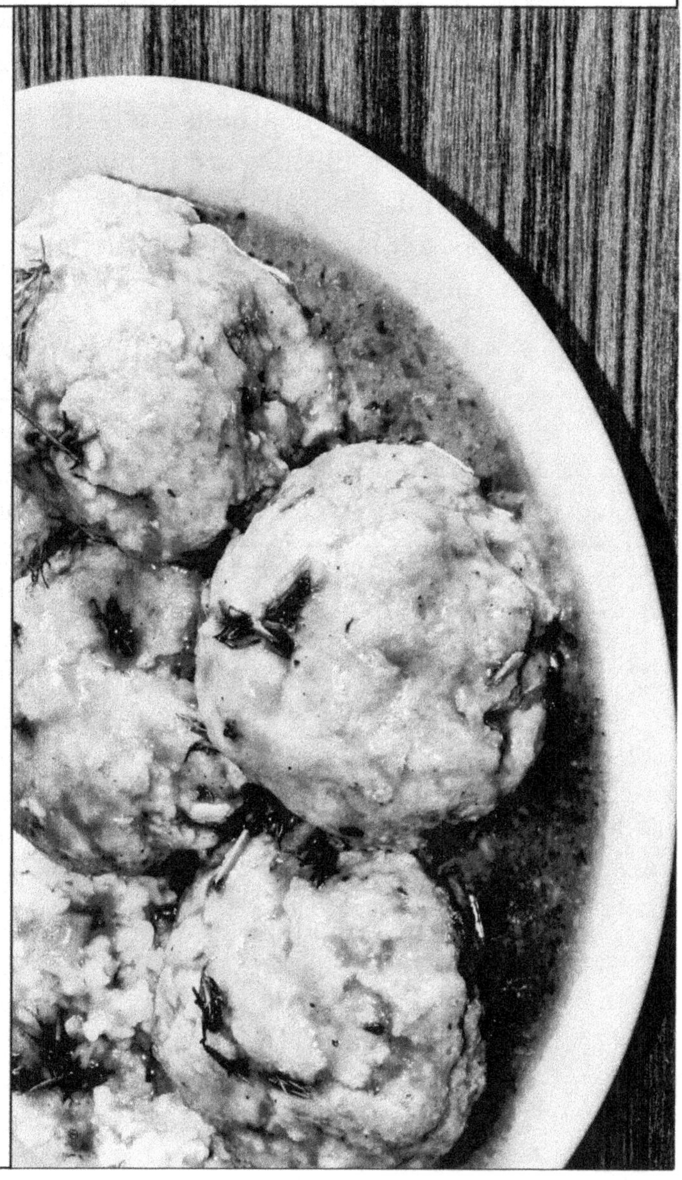

DIRECTIONS:

- In a large sauté pan, heat one tablespoon of oil over medium heat. Add the onions and fennel and cook for 2 to 3 minutes, or until slightly softened. Remove from the heat and set aside to cool.

- In a large mixing bowl, combine the pork, eggs, parsley, fennel seed, salt and pepper. Once the sautéed onions and fennel have cooled, add them to the bowl and mix all the ingredients together with your hands.

- Shape the pork mixture into small meatballs, about 1 ½ inches in diameter. Use a cookie scoop to make sure they are all the same size. Place the meatballs on a parchment-lined baking tray or large plate.

- Wipe the sauté pan clean and add 3 tablespoons of oil over medium heat. Place the first batch of meatballs in the pan, making sure not to overcrowd it (about 20 meatballs).

- Cook the meatballs for 2 to 3 minutes on one side, then rotate them so that all sides are browned. The meatballs should cook for 10 to 12 minutes total, or until the inside is no longer pink. When the first batch is done, remove them to a paper towel-lined plate and start the next batch.

- Discard any fat from the pan and add all of the meatballs back to the pan to warm through before serving.

NOTES:

- If you can't locate ground fennel seed, you can grind it yourself. Simply put the whole seeds in a spice or coffee grinder, or put them in a plastic bag and pound them with a rolling pin or hammer until finely ground.

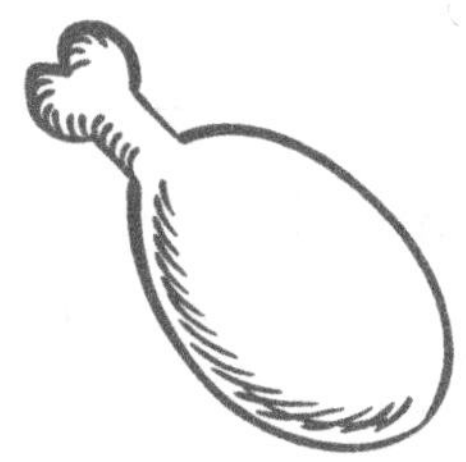

Pesto Chicken

 **PREP TIME:** 10mins	 **COOK TIME:** 10mins	 **SERVINGS:** 6	 **COURSE:** Main Course

Nutritional Value:

Calories: 245.8kcal	Fat: 13.3g	Carb: 4.6g	Protein: 25.7g

INGREDIENTS:

- 1.5 lb chicken breast cutlets
- Salt and Pepper
- Extra virgin olive oil
- 1 zucchini cut into half moons
- 1 red bell pepper cored and cut into strips
- ½ red onion sliced
- 1 cup about 5 oz grape tomatoes
- ⅓ cup basil pesto (homemade or store-bought)
- ⅓ cup cream
- Juice of ½ lemon
- Zest of 1 lemon
- Toasted pine nuts for garnish optional
- Fresh basil for garnish optional

DIRECTIONS:

- Pat chicken breast cutlets dry and season both sides with salt & pepper. (To get thinner pieces, cut boneless skinless chicken breasts in half horizontally. learn the video to learn how I do it).

- In a large cast iron skillet, heat a small amount of extra virgin olive oil (approximately 2 tablespoons) until shimmering but not smoking. Cook the chicken in the skillet for 2 to 3 minutes on each side, flipping once, over medium-high heat. Remove from the skillet and leave aside for the time being.

- Add a little more extra virgin olive oil to the skillet if necessary. Combine the zucchini, bell peppers, onion, and grape tomatoes in a mixing bowl. Season with kosher salt and freshly ground black pepper to taste. Cook, stirring periodically, for 6 to 7 minutes, or until the vegetables have softened.

- Combine the basil pesto and cream in a small bowl or glass measuring cup.

- Return the chicken to the skillet. Pour in the pesto-cream mixture. Reduce the heat to mediumlow and cook for about a minute.

- Remove the skillet from the heat and stir in the lemon juice and zest. Garnish with pine nuts and fresh basil. Serve hot with your favorite grain pasta or plain orzo.

NOTES:

- Chicken breast cutlets are simply boneless, skinless chicken breasts cut in half horizontally to thin them out for even and speedy cooking. If you can't find chicken breast cutlets, use chicken breast meat and cut it in half as directed.

- To serve with your favorite pasta, increase or triple the amount of basil pesto and cream mixture to produce a little extra sauce.

- Leftovers can be stored in the fridge in a tightly sealed container for about 2 nights. You can warm it briefly on the stovetop over medium-low heat (you may need to add a little liquid to assist it).

FRUITS AND SNACKS
RECIPES

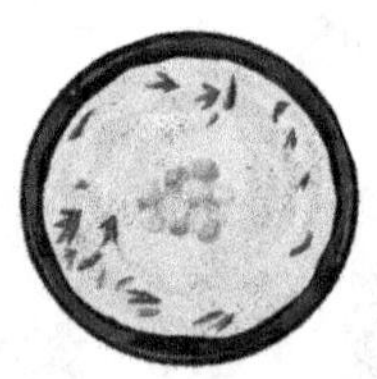 # Green Goddess Hummus

 **PREP TIME:** 5mins	 **COOK TIME:** 0min	 **SERVINGS:** 16 servings	 **COURSE:** Appetizer

Nutritional Value:	Calories: 167kcal	Fat: 1g	Carb: 18g	Protein: 6g

INGREDIENTS:

- 30 oz canned chickpeas (garbanzo beans), drained with liquid reserved (I use two 15oz
- cans)
- 1/3 cup chickpea liquid, or more, as needed
- 1/2 cup tahini
- 1/4 cup olive oil
- 1 cup spinach, moderately packed
- 1/2 cup roughly chopped parsley or other herbs
- 2 lemons, juiced
- 1 green onion, roughly chopped
- 1 clove garlic
- 1 teaspoon cumin
- 1/2 teaspoon salt

GARNISH

- olive oil, chopped herbs, chopped walnuts and sesame seeds

DIRECTIONS:

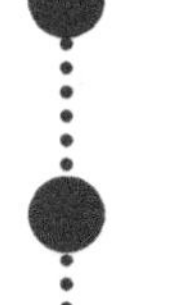 Fill your Vitamix or high-powered blender with all of the ingredients and secure the cover. Insert the tamper after removing the lid cover.

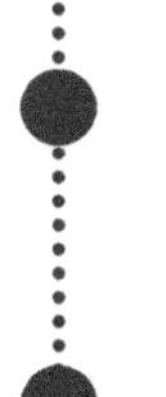 Turn the blender to high for 30 seconds (or longer for a creamier texture) and push the hummus into the blades with the tamper. If you want a softer hummus, add additional chickpea liquid (aquafaba).

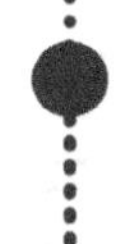 Place the hummus on a serving plate and top with olive oil, herbs, walnuts, and sesame seeds.

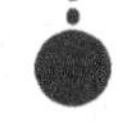 If you want additional herb flavor, feel free to add extra herbs.

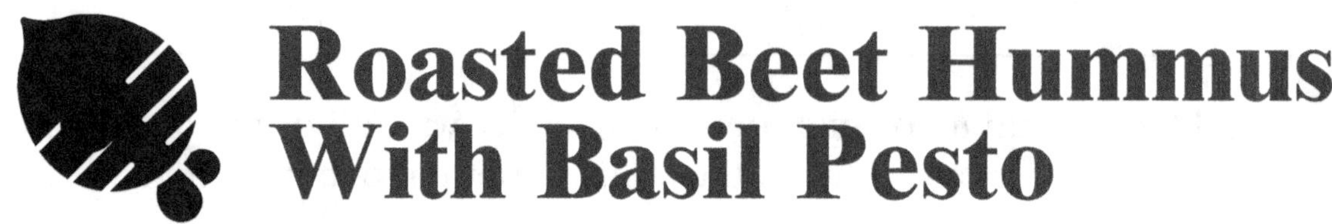

Roasted Beet Hummus With Basil Pesto

 **PREP TIME:** 10mins	 **COOK TIME:** 1hr	 **SERVINGS:** 16 servings	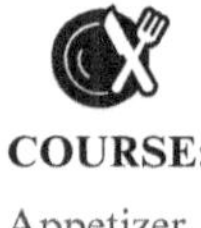 **COURSE:** Appetizer

Nutritional Value:	Calories: 130kcal	Fat: 8g	Carb: 11g	Protein: 4g

INGREDIENTS:

- 2 medium beet
- 2 (15-ounce cans) chickpeas, drained with liquid reserved
- ⅓ cup chickpea liquid , or more, as needed for a smoother consistency
- ½ cup tahini
- ¼ cup olive oil
- 2 lemons, juiced
- 1 clove garlic
- ½ teaspoon salt

GARNISH

- Basil Pesto
- Parsley
- Olive Oil

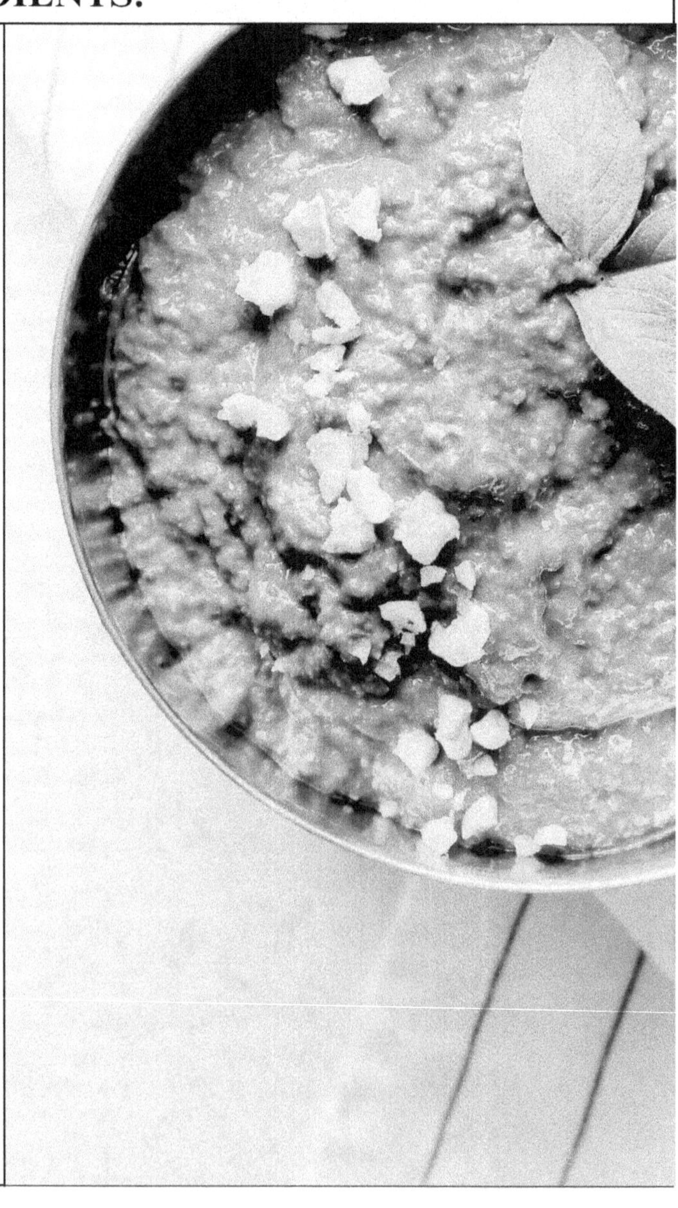

DIRECTIONS:

- Preheat the oven to 400 degrees F.

- Remove the leafy stems from the beets, leaving about 2 inches attached. Wash the beets, lightly coat in olive oil (or avocado oil), and roast for 50 to 60 minutes in a covered cast-iron pot or other baking dish.

- Remove the beets from the oven and snip off the tail and stem

- In a Vitamix or other high-powered blender, combine the chickpeas, chickpea liquid, tahini, lemon juice, olive oil, garlic, salt, and beets. Blend for one minute, or until smooth and creamy, using the tamper.

- Transfer the beet hummus to a serving bowl and top with basil pesto, parsley, and olive oil drizzle.

NOTES:

- The recipe yields around 4 cups of beet hummus. 1/4 cup is the serving size.

Roasted Cauliflower Hummus

			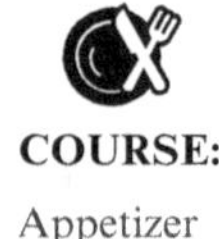
PREP TIME: 10mins	**COOK TIME:** 20mins	**SERVINGS:** 4 servings	**COURSE:** Appetizer

Nutritional Value:	Calories: 235.4kcal	Fat: 18.9g	Carb: 14.7g	Protein: 6.7g

INGREDIENTS:

- 1 large head cauliflower, approx 5 cups florets
- 3 tablespoons olive oil, divided
- ¼ cup tahini
- 2 tablespoons water, or more for desired consistency
- 1 lemon, juiced
- 1 garlic clove
- ¼ teaspoon salt
- ¼ teaspoon ground cumin
- pinch ground coriander
- pepper, to taste
- garnish with olive oil, sunflower seeds and chopped parsley

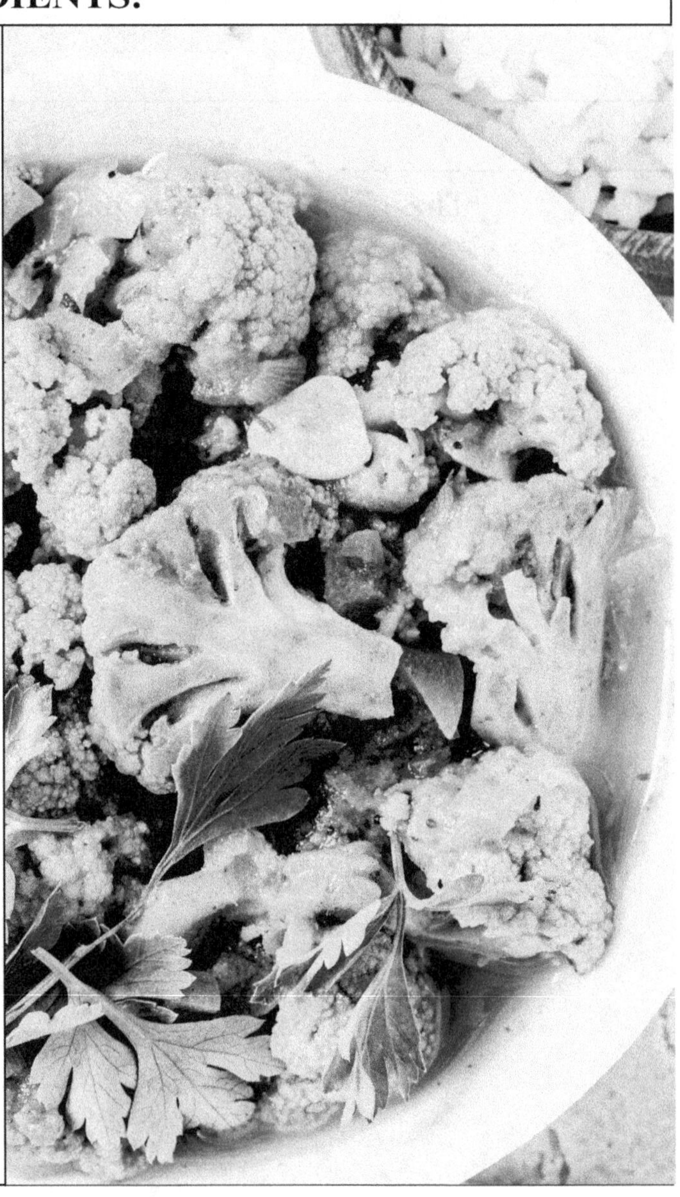

DIRECTIONS:

- Preheat the oven to 400 degrees F.

- Remove the cauliflower florets and lay them on a baking sheet. Toss with 1 tablespoon olive oil (or avocado oil) to mix. Roast the baking tray in the oven for 20 minutes.

- Place the cauliflower in a food processor or Vitamix. Combine the tahini, remaining 2 tablespoons olive oil, water, lemon juice, garlic clove, salt, cumin, and coriander in a mixing bowl. Season with pepper to taste. On high, blend until smooth and creamy.

- Transfer to a serving dish and top with sunflower seeds and parsley

NOTES:

- I enjoy cooking hummus in my Vitamix since it is very creamy. On this recipe, you may need to scrape down the sides of the Vitamix container. That's when I pulled out my under blade scraper!

- If your cauliflower hummus is too thick, simply add more water (a teaspoon at a time) until it reaches the ideal smoothness.

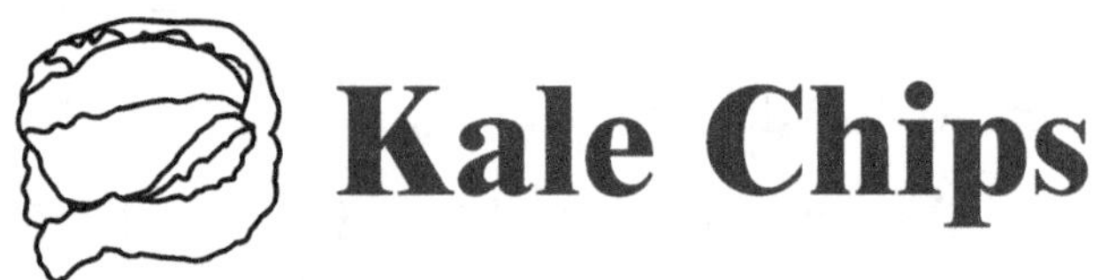

Kale Chips

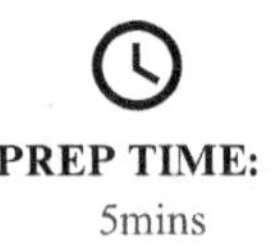			
PREP TIME: 5mins	**COOK TIME:** 10mins	**SERVINGS:** 4 servings	**COURSE:** Appetizer

Nutritional Value:	Calories: 29kcal	Fat: 2g	Carb: 3g	Protein: 2g

INGREDIENTS:	***HEAVY DUTY BAKING SHEET REQUIRED***

- 4 kale stems
- 1 to 2 teaspoons extra virgin olive oil
- ¼ teaspoon kosher salt

DIRECTIONS:

- Remove the kale leaves from the stem. Preheat the oven to 300 degrees Fahrenheit (150 degrees Celsius). Kale should be washed and dried thoroughly. Remove the kale leaves from the stems and shred into bite-sized pieces. In a mixing basin, combine the torn kale.

- Taking kale leaves from the stem.

- In a medium mixing bowl, combine the olive oil, lemon juice, garlic, salt, and pepper. Drizzle the dressing over the Kamut and sprinkle with the feta and dill sprigs to decorate.

- Kale is being massaged with oil and salt

- Cook the kale. Cook the kale in a single layer on a baking pan for 8 minutes. Cook for an additional 2 to 6 minutes, rotating the baking sheet halfway through, monitoring every minute or two to ensure it's not burning.

- Uncooked kale leaves on a baking sheet.

- Allow time for rest. Remove the baking sheet from the oven and set aside for 3 to 5 minutes to cool before serving.

- Kale chips baked on a baking pan.

- These oven-baked kale chips are the ideal healthy snack for any salty, savory, or crunchy craving.

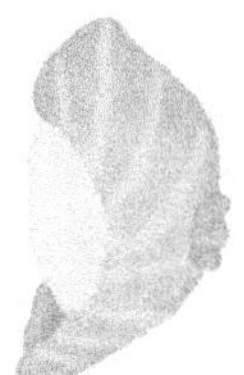

Smoked Salmon, Avocado, And Cucumber Bites

 PREP TIME: 10mins	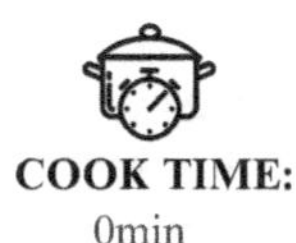 COOK TIME: 0min	 SERVINGS: 12 bites	 COURSE: Appetizer

Nutritional Value:	Calories: 46kcal	Fat: 3g	Carb: 2g	Protein: 3g

INGREDIENTS:

- 1 medium cucumber
- 1 large avocado, peeled and pit removed
- 1/2 tbsp lime juice
- 6 oz smoked salmon
- chives, for garnish
- black pepper, for garnish

DIRECTIONS:

- Cut the cucumber into 1/4-inch slices and arrange them on a plate. In a bowl, mash the avocado and lime juice together with a fork until it's creamy. Then, spread a bit of the avocado mixture on each cucumber slice and top with a thin slice of smoked salmon.

- Finally, sprinkle some finely chopped chives and cracked black pepper on top of each bite. Serve right away!

- These smoked salmon, avocado, and cucumber snacks are a great way to start a meal.

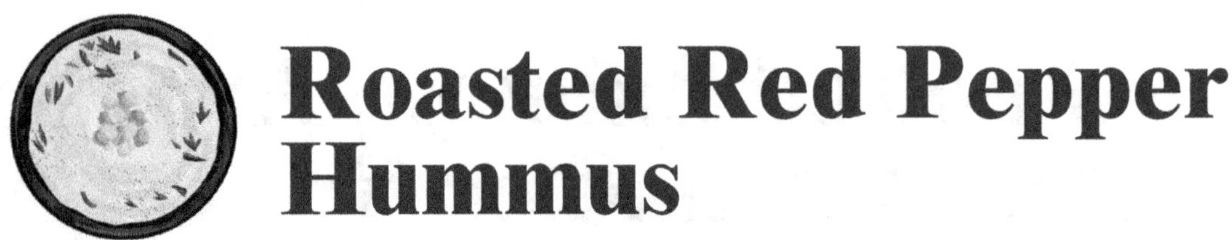

Roasted Red Pepper Hummus

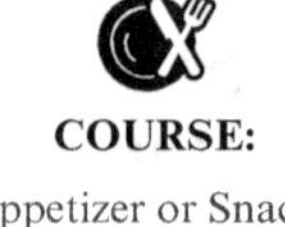

PREP TIME: 5mins	**COOK TIME:** 0min	**SERVINGS:** 16 servings	**COURSE:** Appetizer or Snack

Nutritional Value:	Calories: 169kcal	Fat: 9g	Carb: 18g	Protein: 6g

INGREDIENTS:

- 2 (15-ounce cans) chickpeas (garbanzo beans), drained with liquid reserved
- 1 (16-ounce jar) roasted red peppers, drained and extra liquid removed from peppers
- ½ cup tahini
- ¼ cup aquafaba/chickpea liquid
- ¼ cup olive oil
- 2 lemons, juiced
- 1 garlic clove
- 1 teaspoon cumin
- ½ teaspoon salt

GARNISH

- white sesame seeds
- black sesame seeds
- diced roasted red pepper

DIRECTIONS:

- Fill your Vitamix with all of the ingredients and secure the cover. Insert the tamper after removing the lid cover. Blend the hummus for 30 seconds on high, using the tamper to press it into the blades. If you want a smoother consistency, add additional chickpea juice.

- In a blender, combine the roasted red pepper hummus.

- Serve the hummus with diced roasted red pepper and white and black sesame seeds on top.

NOTES:

- With only a few ingredients, you can prepare roasted red pepper hummus at home. It's flavorful, creamy, smooth, and slightly smokey.

- For a milder flavor, reduce the amount of roasted red peppers in the hummus. Personally, I enjoy it with a strong flavor!

- If you want to put some chopped roasted red pepper on top, save half of a pepper from the blender. Then finely cut it to sprinkle on top.

- If kept in a sealed container, the hummus will keep in the fridge for up to a week. You may also store the hummus in the freezer for later use. This recipe is ideal for meal preparation!

- Don't forget that you can make your own tahini - it's incredibly simple! Simply make my tahini recipe.

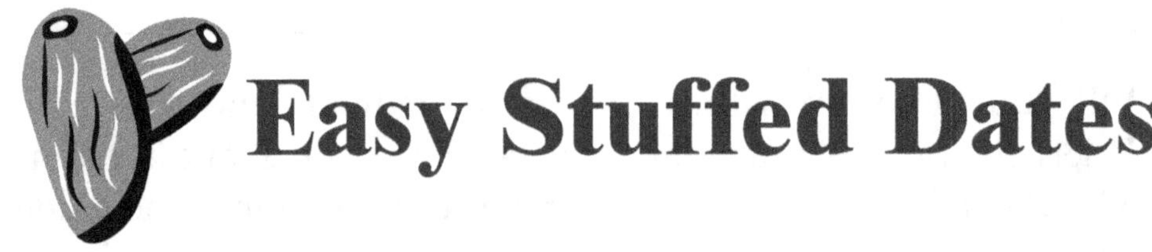

Easy Stuffed Dates

PREP TIME:	COOK TIME:	SERVINGS:	COURSE:
5mins	10mins	8 people	Appetizer

Nutritional Value:	Calories: 227.5kcal	Fat: 5.5g	Carb: 45.5g	Protein: 4.3g

INGREDIENTS:

- 20 large medjool dates
- For Goat Cheese Stuffed Dates:
- 4 ounces goat cheese, at room temperature
- ¼ to ⅓ cup walnut pieces
- Warmed honey, for garnish
- Red pepper flakes, or Aleppo pepper, optional for garnish

DIRECTIONS:

- Cut the cucumber into 1/4-inch slices and arrange them on a plate. In a bowl, mash the avocado and lime juice together with a fork until it's creamy. Then, spread a bit of the avocado mixture on each cucumber slice and top with a thin slice of smoked salmon.

- Finally, sprinkle some finely chopped chives and cracked black pepper on top of each bite. Serve right away!

- These smoked salmon, avocado, and cucumber snacks are a great way to start a meal.

NOTES:

- To serve hot: Preheat the oven to 350 degrees Fahrenheit. Place the pitted dates on a large sheet pan and fill with the goat cheese and walnuts (save the honey for later). Bake for 5 to 10 minutes, or until the dates have softened and warmed through, and the cheese has browned. Finish with honey and pepper flakes after removing from the oven. Serve right away.

- Prepare ahead of time: You can make these goat cheese stuffed dates a day or two ahead of time. Simply place them on a plate in a single layer in the fridge. Remove them from the oven and set them aside to cool to room temperature before serving.

- If you are unable to use honey, substitute our fig jam. Simply thin it with a little water and drizzle it over the dates.

Other topping options....

- Manchego cheese and sliced Granny Smith apples with a dollop of fig jam (our Greek fig jam is a great choice!) is a delicious combination.

- If you're looking for something a bit different, try peanut butter and almond butter or tahini with chocolate chips.

- For a savory snack, stuff dates with feta cheese, sun-dried tomatoes, basil chiffonade, and a sprinkle of red pepper flakes (Aleppo pepper is a great option).

- Or, if you're looking for something simpler, just stuff your dates with almonds, walnuts, or cashews - no need to chop them! Just pop them right inside the dates.

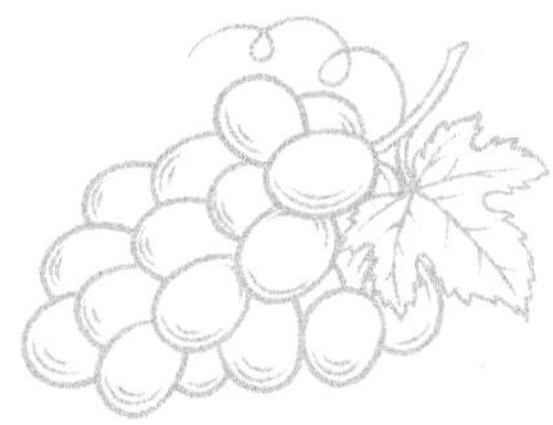

Roasted Grape Crostini with Ricotta Honey

 **PREP TIME:** 5mins	 **COOK TIME:** 30mins	 **SERVINGS:** 12 - 14 Crostini	 **COURSE:** Appetizer

Nutritional Value:	Calories: 174kcal	Fat: 5.1g	Carb: 26.5g	Protein: 6.3g

INGREDIENTS:

For the crostini

- 12-14 slices of baguette
- olive oil

For the roasted grapes

- 2 cups red grapes
- 1 1/2 tbsp balsamic vinegar
- 1 1/2 tbsp olive oil
- 1/4 tsp salt
- 1/4 tsp ground pepper

For the ricotta

- 1 cup ricotta
- zest of one lemon
- 2 tbsp honey
- fresh thyme or rosemary for garnish

DIRECTIONS:

For the crostini

- Heat the oven to 400F. Cut the baguette into 1-inch thick slices, about 12-14 of them, using a bread knife. Spread olive oil on one side of the baguette slices and arrange them in a single layer on a baking sheet. Bake for 10 minutes, flipping the slices halfway through. Once done, set aside.

For the roasted grapes

- While the crostini is baking, prepare the grapes by tossing the grapes with balsamic vinegar, olive oil, salt, and pepper on a sheet pan lined with parchment paper.

- When the crostini is done, bake the grapes in the oven for 15-17 minutes, or until softened and the grapes begin to burst. Allow the grapes to cool for a few minutes before assembling the crostini.

For the ricotta

- Set aside the ricotta, lemon zest, and honey.

- Spread about 1 tbsp of the ricotta mixture on each crostini, top with a few grapes, and garnish with a sprig of fresh thyme or rosemary

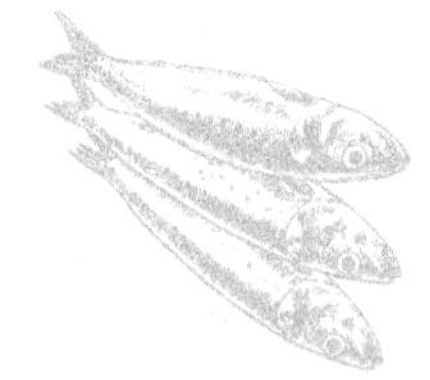

Sardine Salad Crackers

PREP TIME: 15mins	**COOK TIME:** 5mins	**SERVINGS:** 4 people	**COURSE:** Lunch

Nutritional Value:	Calories: 235kcal	Fat: 14g	Carb: 6g	Protein: 23g

INGREDIENTS:

- 8 sardine fillets, canned or fresh
- 4 cups mixed salad greens
- 1 cup cherry tomatoes, halved
- 1/2 cup kalamata olives, pitted
- Salt and pepper to taste
- 1/4 cup red onion, thinly sliced
- 2 tablespoons capers
- 2 tablespoons fresh lemon juice
- 2 tablespoons extra virgin olive oil

DIRECTIONS:

- Preheat a grill or grill pan to medium-high heat.
- Season both sides of the sardine fillets with salt and pepper.
- Grill the sardine fillets for 2-3 minutes per side, or until done and slightly browned. Set aside after removing from the heat.
- Combine the mixed salad greens, cherry tomatoes, kalamata olives, red onion, and capers in a large salad bowl.
- Whisk together the lemon juice and olive oil in a small bowl. Season with salt and pepper to taste.
- Toss the salad with the dressing to mix it.
- Serve the salad on plates, topped with 2 grilled sardine fillets.
- Serve right away.

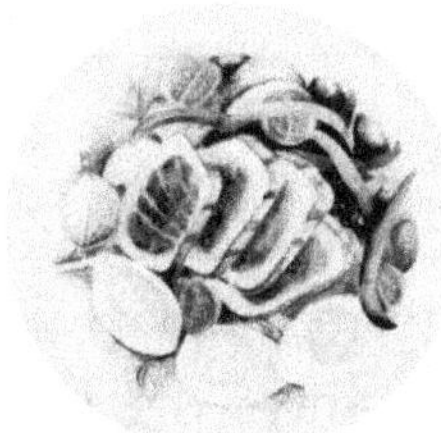

Tuna Salad Spread

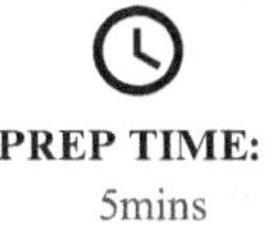 **PREP TIME:** 5mins	 **COOK TIME:** 0min	 **SERVINGS:** 4	 **COURSE:** Appetizer or Snack

Nutritional Value:	Calories: 130kcal	Fat: 8g	Carb: 6g	Protein: 10g

INGREDIENTS:

- 1 avocado, mashed
- 2 tablespoons low-fat plain Greek yogurt
- 1 tablespoon lemon juice
- 1 tablespoon chopped fresh parsley
- ¼ teaspoon garlic powder
- ¼ teaspoon paprika
- ¼ teaspoon salt
- ¼ teaspoon ground pepper
- 1 (5 ounce) can albacore tuna in water, drained
- ¼ cup diced onion or celery

DIRECTIONS:

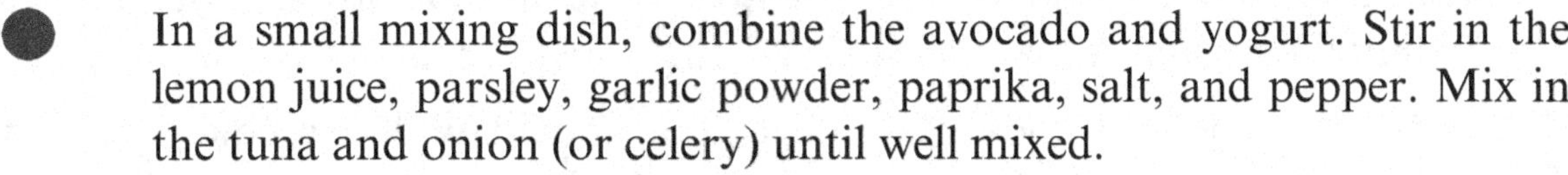

- In a small mixing dish, combine the avocado and yogurt. Stir in the lemon juice, parsley, garlic powder, paprika, salt, and pepper. Mix in the tuna and onion (or celery) until well mixed.

NOTES:

- How to Make a Delicious Tuna Salad Spread.

- Tuna salad spread is typically made with mayonnaise, tuna, and little else. However, not this one! Instead, we take a lighter approach and spice up a plain can of tuna with mashed avocado and Greek yogurt. Here's how we made this tuna spread more nutritious:

- Remove the mayonnaise

- Mayonnaise functions as a binder in tuna salad spread, holding everything together and imparting a creamy texture. It also provides a substantial amount of calories and saturated fat. We omitted the mayonnaise entirely in favor of a blend of mashed avocado and low-fat Greek yogurt.

- The avocado contains a lot of monounsaturated fat, which is a good fat that can help lower "bad" LDL cholesterol and lower the risk of heart disease and stroke. A dash of low-fat Greek yogurt adds sharpness (along with a squeeze of lemon juice) and smoothness akin to mayonnaise, but with fewer saturated fat and calories.

- Use High-Quality Tuna

- For our tuna salad spread, we use albacore tuna packed in water. Albacore tuna is light, solid, and mild, and it is high in Omega-3 fatty acids. Tuna in water contains fewer calories and fat than tuna in oil. When shopping for good tuna, read the label to ensure that the can only includes water, tuna, and salt and no other additives. Look for free school, pole-and-linecaught, school-caught, troll-caught, or FAD-free on the label to locate a sustainable option. For additional information on sustainable seafood options, visit the Monterey Bay Aquarium Seafood Watch.

What Should You Serve With Tuna Salad Spread?

- You can eat healthy tuna salad on a sandwich, in a wrap, or on whole-wheat crackers. Tuna salad spread can be stuffed into halves small peppers, celery sticks, sliced cucumber, or lettuce leaves.

- We recommend consuming this tuna spread within a few hours of creating it since it contains avocado, which can brown quickly. It only takes 5 minutes from start to finish, so making a fresh batch whenever you need it is quick and simple.

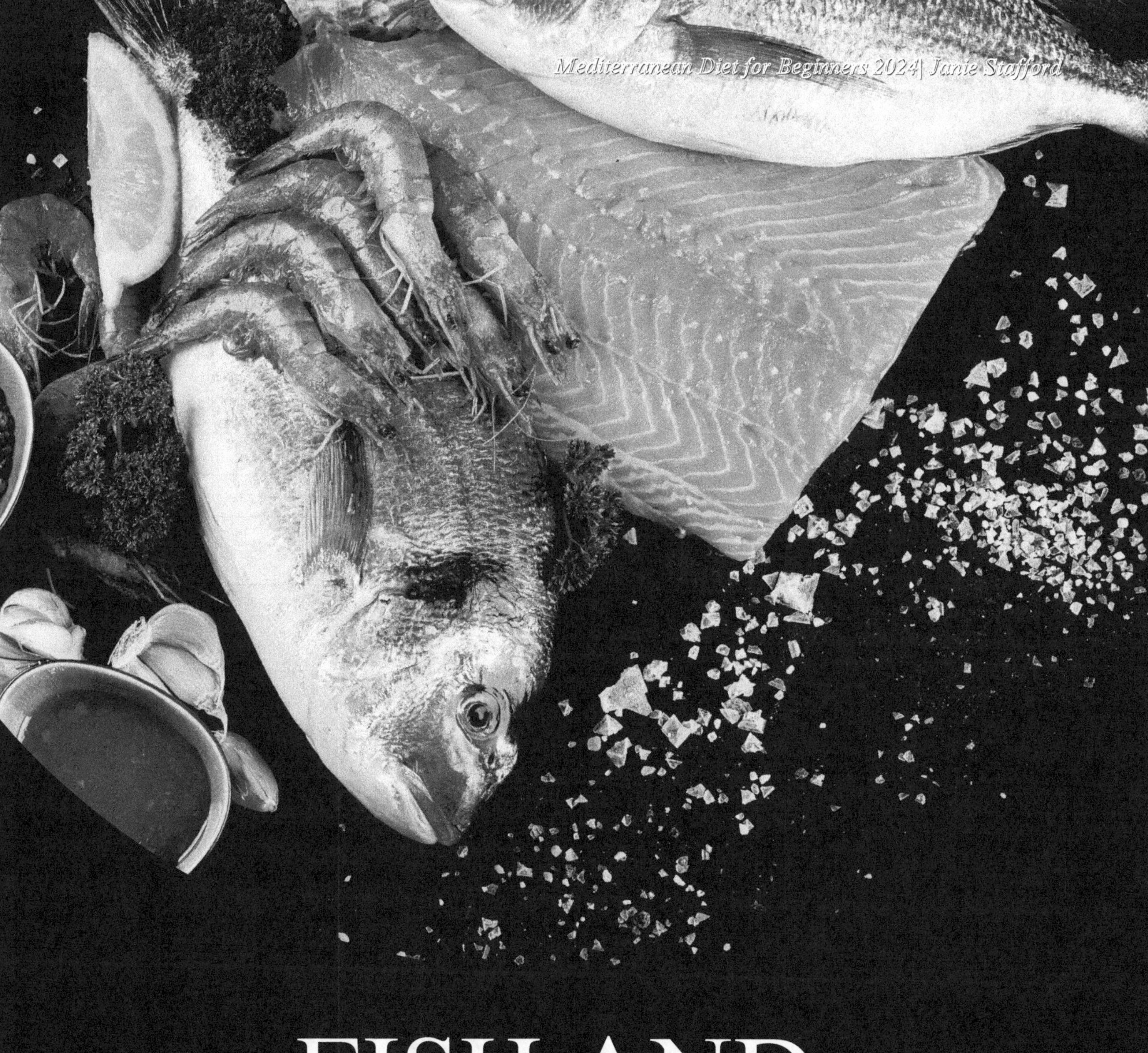

FISH AND SEAFOOD

RECIPES

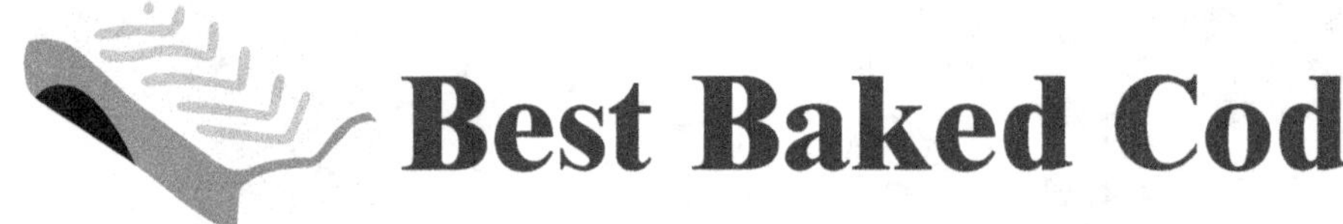

Best Baked Cod

 **PREP TIME:** 10mins	 **COOK TIME:** 15mins	 **SERVINGS:** 4 servings	 **COURSE:** Main Course

Nutritional Value:	Calories: 258kcal	Fat: 13g	Carb: 4g	Protein: 31g

INGREDIENTS:

- 4 (6-ounce) cod filets
- 3 tablespoons butter, softened
- 1 tablespoon extra virgin olive oil
- 3 garlic cloves, minced
- 2 tablespoons parsley, chives, thyme or other herbs, finely chopped
- ½ teaspoon paprika
- 1 lemon, thinly sliced
- kosher salt and freshly ground black pepper, to taste

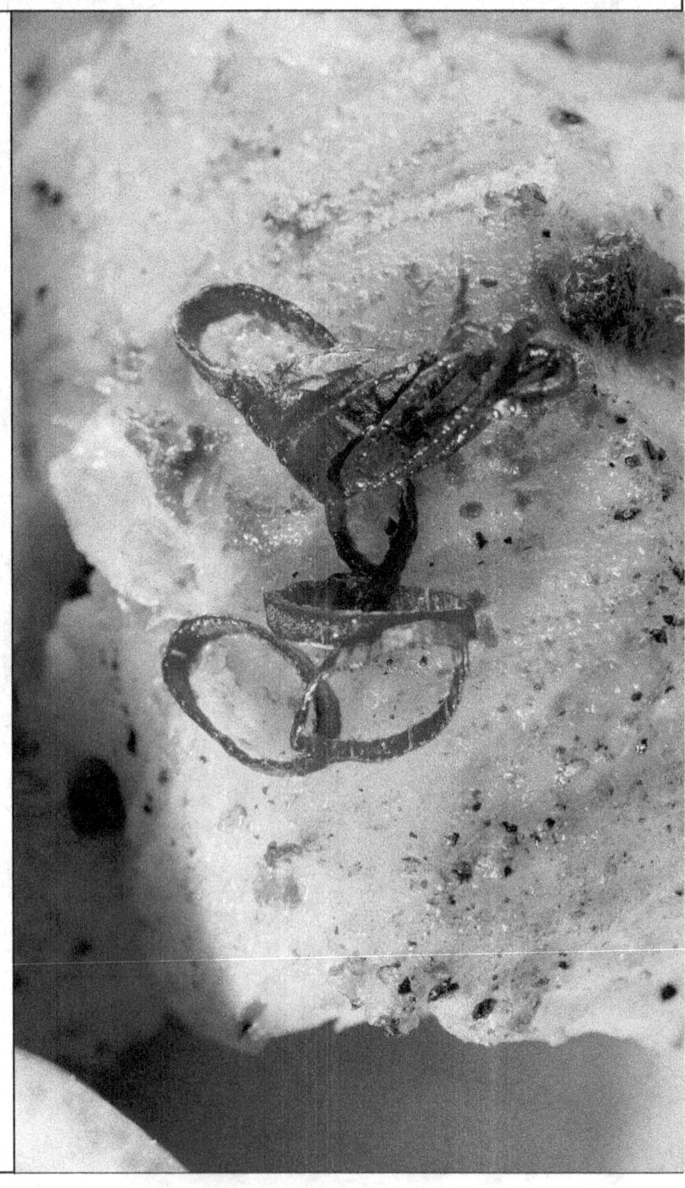

DIRECTIONS:

- Preheat the oven to 400 degrees Fahrenheit (200 degrees Celsius). Fill a baking dish halfway with cod

  <u>Four cod fillets in a baking dish.</u>
- Combine the butter, olive oil, minced garlic, parsley, paprika, salt, and pepper in a small mixing bowl.

  <u>Mixing the garlic herb butter mixture.</u>
  - Top each filet with the compound butter mixture.
  - Cod fillets in garlic herb butter.
  - Place the lemon slices on top and underneath the fish filets.
  - Lemon slices on top of cod fillets.
  - Bake for 13 to 15 minutes, or until the fish is opaque and readily flaked with a fork. Before
  - serving, ladle the baking dish juices over the cod.
  - Cod baked in a baking dish.

NOTES:

- This baked cod recipe is simple and straightforward, yielding deliciously buttery, garlicky, and flaky fish every time!

  <u>EQUIPMENT</u>
- Casserole Dish This pan can hold multiple fish fillets!

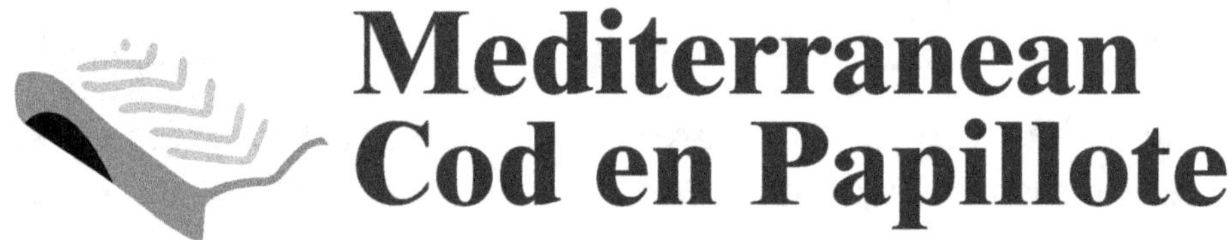

Mediterranean Cod en Papillote

 **PREP TIME:** 15mins	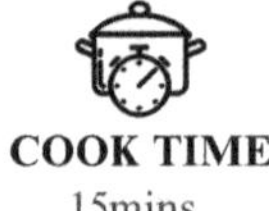 **COOK TIME:** 15mins	 **SERVINGS:** 4 servings	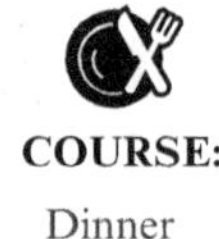 **COURSE:** Dinner

Nutritional Value:	Calories: 275kcal	Fat: 12g	Carb: 12g	Protein: 33g

INGREDIENTS:

- 1 medium zucchini
- 4 (6-ounce) cod filets
- kosher salt and freshly ground black pepper, to taste
- 2 lemons, thinly sliced
- 1 small shallot, thinly sliced
- 4 sprigs fresh thyme
- 20 olives, halved or quartered
- 20 grape tomatoes, halved
- 2 tablespoons extra-virgin olive oil

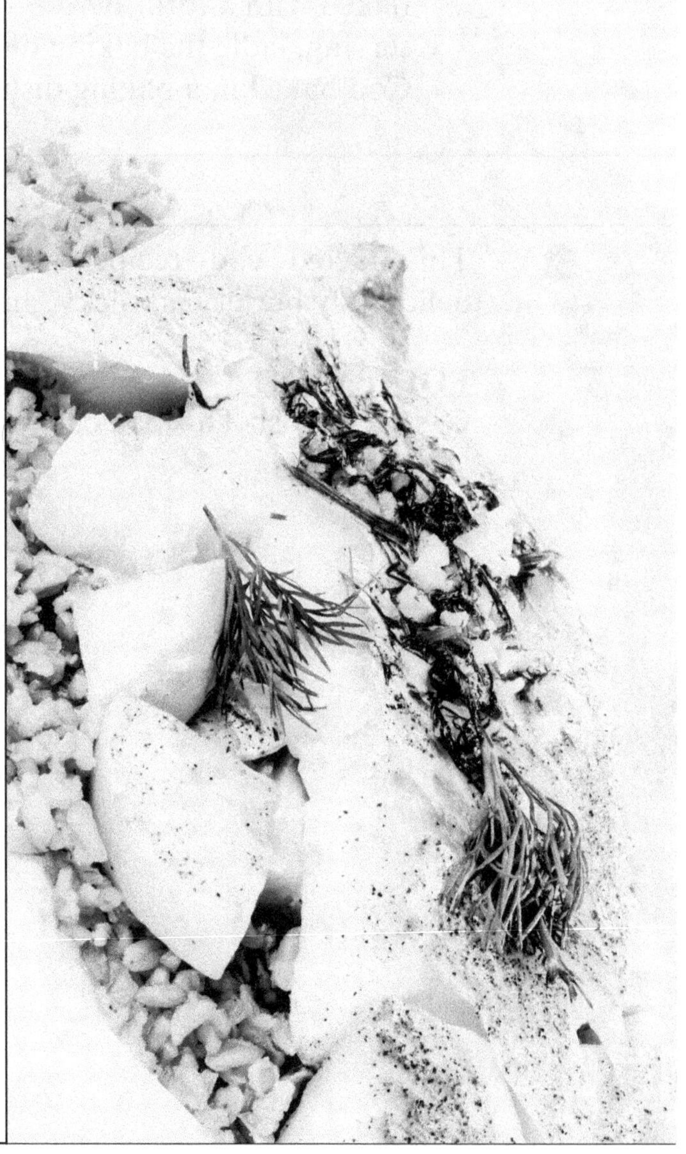

DIRECTIONS:

- Put the packets together. Preheat the oven to 400 degrees Fahrenheit (200 degrees Celsius). Fold a sheet of parchment paper in half and then open it. Place six zucchini slices in the center of one half, then top with a piece of cod. Season with salt and pepper to taste.

- **<u>Prepping cod for fish en papillote</u>**
  Toppings are optional. 2 to 3 lemon slices, a few shallot slices, a sprig of thyme, 5 olives, and 5 tomatoes (it's good if these fall to the side) should be placed on top of the cod. Drizzle some olive oil on top.

- **<u>Adding fish en papillote layers on parchment paper</u>**
  Fold and seal the envelope. Fold the top half of the parchment paper over the bottom half, then tightly wrap up the edges of the parchment paper around the cod. Rep with the last three pieces of cod.

- Making a bag out of a papillote fish

- Bake. Bake the 4 parchment paper packets on a baking sheet for 14 to 18 minutes (depending on thickness), or until the cod is opaque and flakes readily with a fork.

- A baking sheet with en papillote fish

- To provide service. Before serving, pierce the middle of each paper package with a knife and open it up.

NOTES:

- This Mediterranean fish en papillote is the most brilliant way to make a quick, nutritious, and tasty dinner!

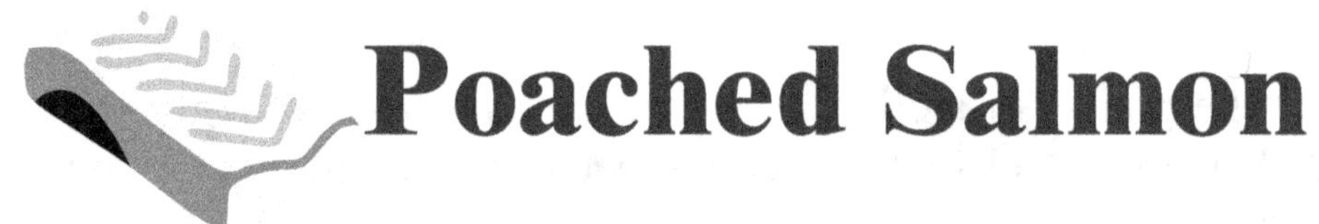

Poached Salmon

 **PREP TIME:** 10mins	 **COOK TIME:** 10mins	 **SERVINGS:** 4 servings	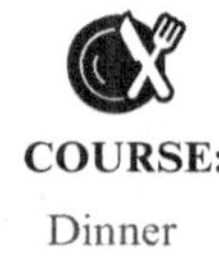 **COURSE:** Dinner

Nutritional Value:	Calories: 268kcal	Fat: 11g	Carb: 6g	Protein: 35g

INGREDIENTS:

- 2 lemons, one thinly sliced for poaching and the other quartered for squeezing on top
- 1 small shallot, thinly sliced
- 3 to 4 sprigs tender fresh herbs (dill, parsley, cilantro, tarragon, etc)
- ½ cup white wine
- ½ cup water
- 4 (6-ounce) salmon filets
- kosher salt and freshly ground black pepper, to taste

DIRECTIONS:

- Make up the poaching liquid. In a large skillet, combine the lemon slices, shallot, fresh herbs, wine, and water. Bring to a low boil over medium heat.

  Making the poaching liquid in the pan
- Mix in the salmon. Season the salmon filets (skin side down) in the pan, cover the pan, and poach for 5 to 7 minutes, depending on the thickness of the salmon.

- Salmon poaching in a pan

- Garnish with parsley and serve. Garnish the poached salmon with fresh herbs and lemon juice. You can even sprinkle hollandaise sauce on top before serving if desired!

- In a pan, poach fish with herbs.

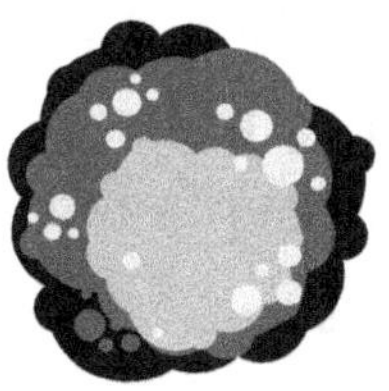

Baked Tuna Meatballs

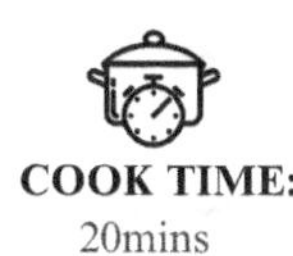
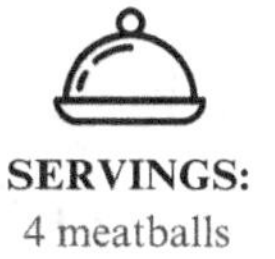

PREP TIME: 20mins	**COOK TIME:** 20mins	**SERVINGS:** 4 meatballs	**COURSE:** Appetizer or Main Course

Nutritional Value:	Calories: 243kcal	Fat: 12g	Carb: 4g	Protein: 28g

INGREDIENTS:

- 1 tablespoon olive oil
- 1/2 medium onion, finely diced
- 2 cups baby spinach, chopped
- 2 cloves garlic, minced
- 3 5-ounce cans tuna, or one pound cooked tuna
- 1/4 cup almond flour
- 2 beaten eggs
- 1 tablespoon mayonnaise
- 1 tablespoon lemon juice
- 2 tablespoons chopped fresh parsley
- 2 tablespoon chopped fresh dill, chopped
- salt and pepper, to taste

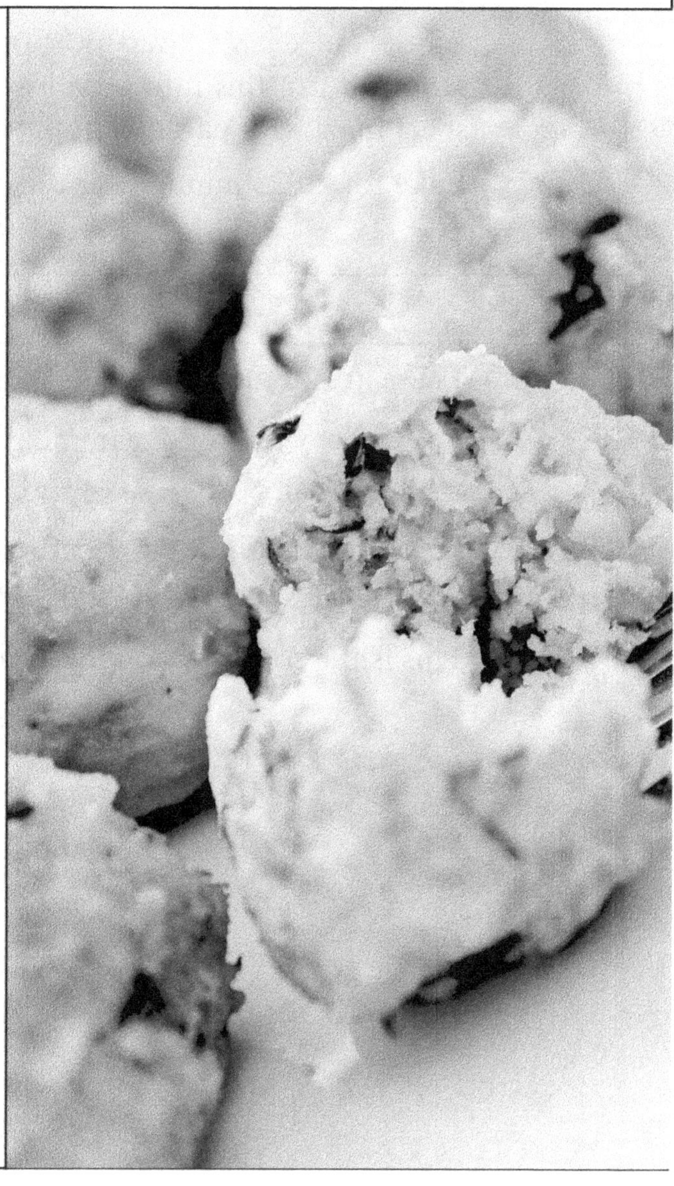

DIRECTIONS:

- In a medium-sized saucepan, heat the oil. Sauté the diced onion and minced garlic for a minute. Then add the chopped baby spinach and cook for another 1-2 minutes, or until wilted.

- Allow the onion spinach combination to cool in a bowl. To expedite the process, place the bowl in the refrigerator.

- Preheat the oven to 400 degrees F.

- Drain the tuna cans and combine them with the cooled veggies, almond flour, eggs, mayonnaise, lemon juice, parsley, dill, salt, and pepper in a mixing bowl.

- Dig in with your hands and stir everything together, breaking up any large bits of tuna. The finer the combination, the simpler it will adhere to one another.

- Scoop out evenly sized portions of mixture using a medium cookie scoop. Form this into a ball with your fingers and lay it on a baking sheet lined with parchment paper.

- Bake for 20-25 minutes, or until the tuna meatballs are faintly brown.

NOTES:

- There are 20 tuna meatballs in this recipe.

- For finicky seafood eaters, this dish is milder in flavor than my salmon patties, so give it a try!

- If your meatballs are too soft, add a bit extra almond flour or coconut flour (both of which are quite absorbent).

- This is the cookie scoop that I use and enjoy.

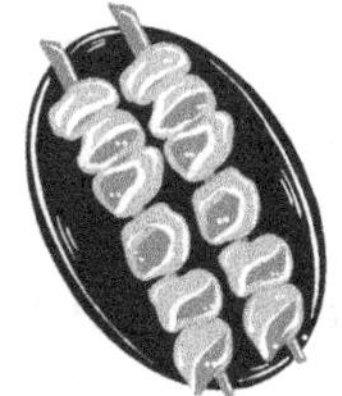

Garlic Grilled Shrimp Skewers

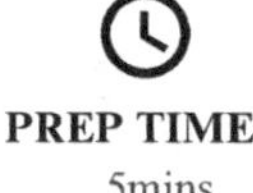 **PREP TIME:** 5mins	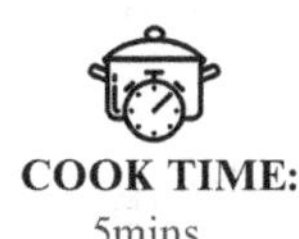 **COOK TIME:** 5mins	 **SERVINGS:** 5 servings	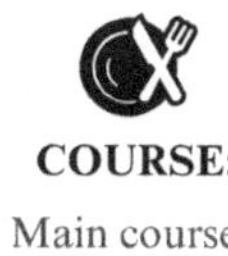 **COURSE:** Main course

Nutritional Value:	Calories: 190kcal	Fat: 2g	Carb: 1g	Protein: 19g

INGREDIENTS:

- 1 pound large shrimp
- 1/4 cup olive oil
- 1/4 cup fresh cilantro, finely chopped
- 1/4 cup fresh parsley, finely chopped
- 4 cloves garlic, minced
- 1 tablespoon lemon juice
- 1/2 teaspoon salt
- 1/4 teaspoon black pepper
- pinch cayenne pepper, adjust to spice preference

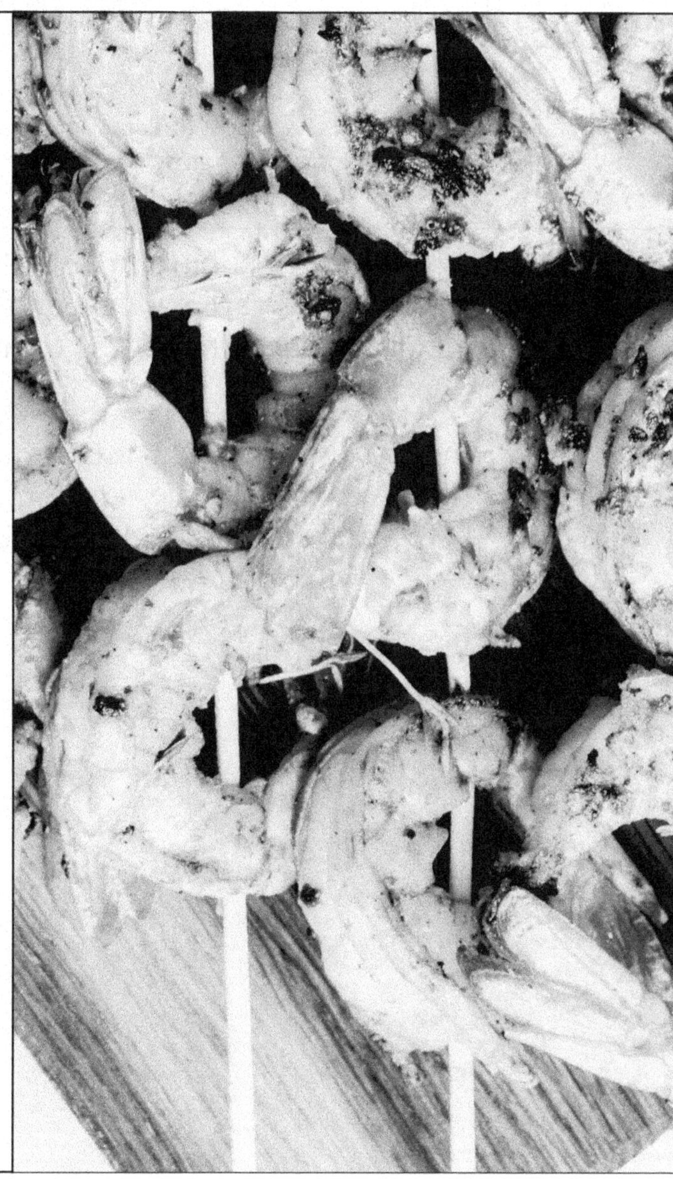

DIRECTIONS:

- In a small mixing bowl, whisk together the olive oil, lemon juice, herbs, garlic, and spices.

- Put the shrimp in a bowl and pour 3/4 of the marinade over them. Gently combine until the shrimp are evenly coated.

- Cover the bowl and leave the shrimp to marinade for 30 minutes to an hour.

- Thread the shrimp onto the skewers, making sure to obtain all of the good garlic and herbs from the bowl and sprinkle them on top of the shrimp.

- On medium high heat, heat a grill or grill pan.

- Once the grill is hot, set the shrimp skewers on it and cook for 2-3 minutes per side, or until the shrimp turn pink and opaque.

- Transfer the shrimp to a platter and drizzle with the leftover marinade before serving.

NOTES:

- Adding the final bit of marinade at the end gives these grilled shrimp an additional garlicky flavor. If you don't like raw garlic and/or want the garlic flavor to be less overpowering, use the entire marinade in step 2.

- In this dish, you can use a variety of fresh herbs, such as parsley, cilantro, basil, thyme, and oregano (I don't recommend rosemary). Feel free to substitute your preferred herbs.

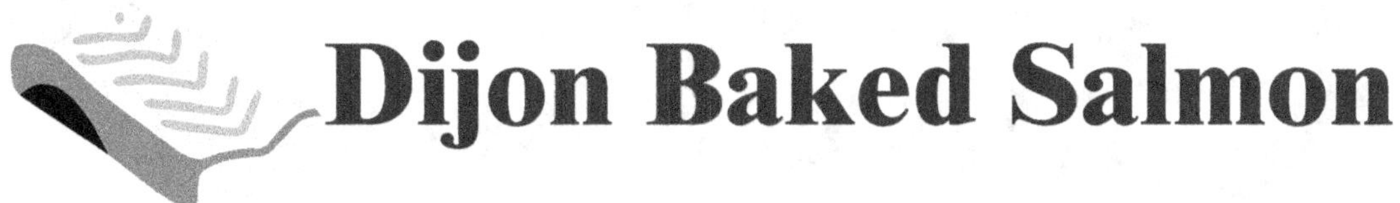

Dijon Baked Salmon

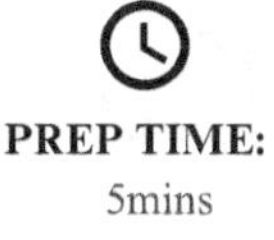			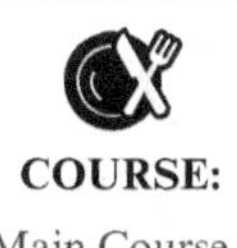
PREP TIME: 5mins	**COOK TIME:** 20mins	**SERVINGS:** 5 servings	**COURSE:** Main Course

Nutritional Value:	Calories: 249.7kcal	Fat: 13.4g	Carb: 1.9g	Protein: 30.5g

INGREDIENTS:

- 1 ½ pounds salmon, King, Sockeye or Coho salmon
- ¼ cup fresh parsley, finely chopped
- ¼ cup Dijon mustard
- 1 tablespoon lemon juice
- 1 tablespoon extra-virgin olive oil
- 3 garlic cloves, finely chopped
- salt and pepper, to taste

DIRECTIONS:

- Preheat the oven to 375 degrees F. In a small bowl, combine the mustard, parsley, lemon juice, oil, garlic, salt, and pepper.
- In a mixing bowl, combine the sauce for the dijon baked salmon.
- Place the salmon on a baking sheet lined with parchment paper and generously cover the top with the herbed mustard mixture.
- Bake the salmon for 18 to 20 minutes (depending on size and thickness), then slice and serve immediately.

NOTES:

- This recipe could easily be made with 4-6 individual salmon fillets instead of one giant fillet.
- If you're doing Whole30, I recommend this Whole30-compliant Dijon mustard. In addition, there are many more Whole30 dishes in the recipe index.
- And if you're searching for some delicious dinner prep ideas, this Dijon baked salmon is always at the top of my list. I'd happily eat this salmon for several days in a row!

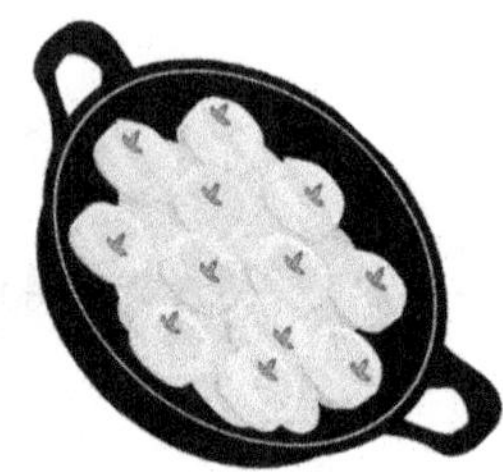

Scallops with Citrus Ginger Sauce

			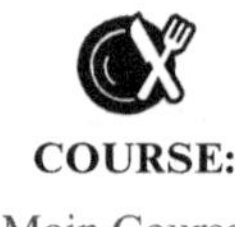
PREP TIME:	**COOK TIME:**	**SERVINGS:**	**COURSE:**
5mins	5mins	4 servings	Main Course

Nutritional Value:	Calories: 254kcal	Fat: 13g	Carb: 12g	Protein: 21g

INGREDIENTS:

- 2 tbsp avocado oil
- 1 1/2 lb sea scallops
- 1 orange, zested and juiced
- 1 lemon, juiced
- 1 tbsp fresh ginger, grated
- 2 tbsp butter, or ghee
- sea salt, to taste
- fresh thyme, for garnish

DIRECTIONS:

- Dry your scallops with a paper towel and season with sea salt.
- In a sauté pan over medium high heat, heat the oil. Place your scallops in the pan when the oil is practically smoking and sear for one and a half to two minutes on each side. Transfer the scallops to a dish.
- Reduce the heat to medium and stir in the orange and lemon juice, orange zest, ginger, and butter. In the pan, whisk together the sauce until it's simmering, then return the scallops to the pan and spoon the sauce on top.
- Plate the scallops, drizzle with additional sauce, and decorate with thyme.

NOTES:

- In this recipe, avocado oil is recommended over olive oil because it is heated nearly to its smoke point. At higher temperatures, avocado oil is more stable.
- Scallops are better slightly undercooked than overcooked. They'll continue to cook after you take them off the heat, just like most meats and fish.

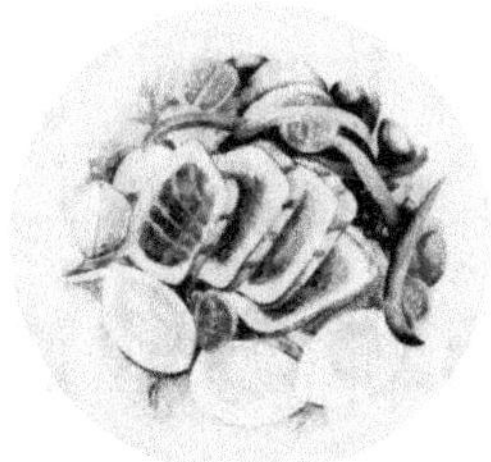

Tuna Salad

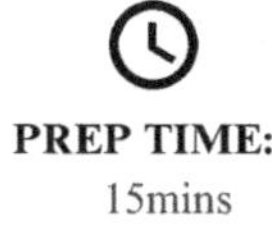	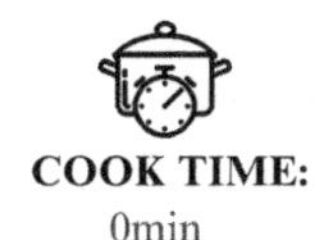		
PREP TIME: 15mins	**COOK TIME:** 0min	**SERVINGS:** 4 servings	**COURSE:** Main Course

Nutritional Value:	Calories: 172kcal	Fat: 11g	Carb: 1g	Protein: 17g

INGREDIENTS:

- 2 (5-ounce) cans tuna
- ¼ cup mayonnaise
- 1 stalk of celery, diced
- 2 tablespoons red onion, diced
- 1-2 tablespoons chopped parsley, chives and/or other herbs
- ½ tablespoon Dijon mustard
- salt and pepper, to taste

DIRECTIONS:

- Remove the tuna cans' liquid. Then, in a mixing dish, combine the tuna, mayonnaise, diced celery, diced red onion, herbs, Dijon mustard, salt, and pepper.
- Tuna salad ingredients in a mixing dish.
- Stir in all of the ingredients until fully blended.
- Tuna salad can be eaten simply, wrapped in lettuce, or as a sandwich.

NOTES:

- You can easily add more mayonnaise if you want a creamier texture.
- Albacore tuna is my favorite, and I always buy Wild Planet brand.

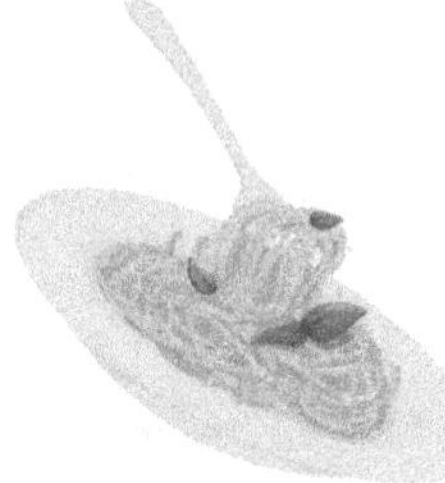

Zucchini Pasta with Lemon Garlic Shrimp

 **PREP TIME:** 10mins	 **COOK TIME:** 5mins	 **SERVINGS:** 4 servings	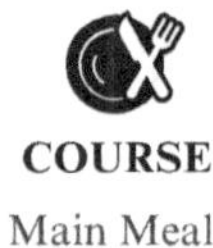 **COURSE:** Main Meal

Nutritional Value:	Calories: 306.2kcal	Fat: 14.5g	Carb: 12.3g	Protein: 27.4g

INGREDIENTS:

- 4 medium zucchini
- 1.5 lb approx 30 raw shrimp, peeled and deveined
- 2 tbsp olive oil
- 4 garlic cloves, finely chopped
- 2 tbsp butter or ghee
- 1 lemon, juice and zest
- 1/4 cup white wine, or chicken broth
- 1/4 cup chopped parsley
- pinch of red pepper flakes
- salt and pepper, to taste

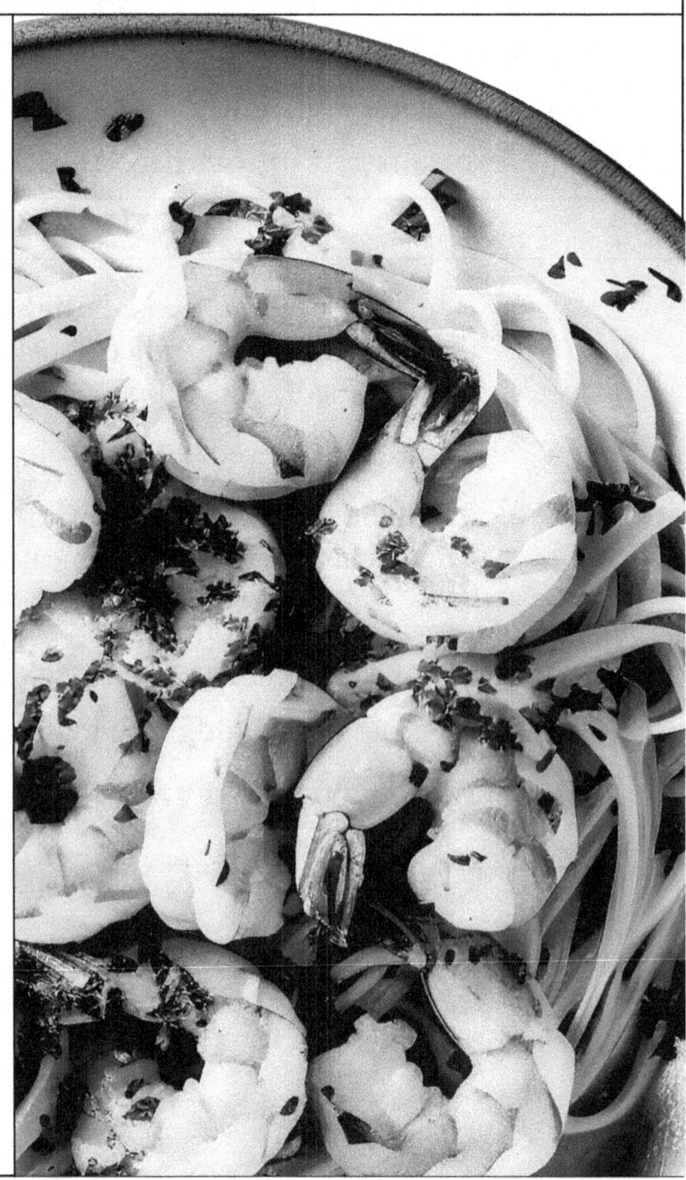

DIRECTIONS:

- Wash the zucchini and trim the ends. Make zucchini pasta with a spiralizer. After that, set aside.

- In a large skillet over medium-high heat, heat the oil. Sprinkle with salt and pepper and arrange the shrimp in a single layer. Cook for one minute, without stirring, to crisp up the bottom side.

- Stir in the garlic, then sauté the shrimp for another minute or two on the other side. Transfer the shrimp to a plate with a large spoon or tongs.

- To the pan, add the butter, lemon juice and zest, red pepper flakes, and white wine. Simmer for 2-3 minutes, stirring occasionally.

- Stir in the parsley, then toss in the zucchini pasta for 30 seconds to reheat it. Return the shrimp to the pan and continue to stir for another minute. Serve right away.

NOTES:

- If you've read my piece on How to Make and Cook Zucchini Noodles, you'll know that I dislike making zucchini noodles. They immediately become limp and wet. So you just want to heat up the zucchini spaghetti without fully cooking it. This preserves the pasta crisp and al dente.

- My 3-Blade Paderno Spiralizer is the spiralizer I use in this dish and all of my vegetarian noodle recipes. But there's also a 6-Blade Paderno Spiralizer!

- I'm frequently asked whether zucchini pasta recipes can be refrigerated and reheated. Unfortunately, because zucchini contains 95% water, these are not the ideal dishes to freeze/reheat once prepared.

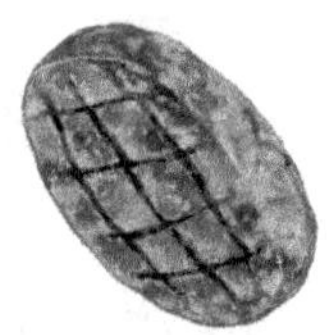

Salmon Patties

PREP TIME: 15mins	**COOK TIME:** 30mins	**SERVINGS:** 2 Patties	**COURSE:** Main Meal

Nutritional Value:

Calories: 243kcal	Fat: 19g	Carb: 6g	Protein: 12g

INGREDIENTS:

- 1 pound fresh salmon
- ⅓ cup olive oil, divided
- 1 medium onion, finely diced
- 1 red bell pepper, finely diced
- 1 to 2 garlic cloves, minced
- ½ cup almond flour
- 2 large eggs, beaten
- 2 tablespoons mayonnaise
- 1 tablespoon Dijon mustard
- ⅓ cup fresh parsley, finely chopped
- 2 tablespoons fresh dill, finely chopped
- kosher salt and black pepper
- LEMON DILL MAYONNAISE (OPTIONAL)
- 1 cup mayonnaise
- 2 tablespoons finely chopped fresh dill
- ½ lemon, zested and juiced (about 1 ½ tablespoons juice)
- kosher salt and black pepper

DIRECTIONS:

- Salmon should be baked. Preheat the oven to 425 degrees Fahrenheit. Drizzle a tablespoon of olive oil over the salmon and season generously with salt and black pepper. Cook for 10 to 13 minutes, or until just done. Then, remove the salmon from the oven and place it in the refrigerator to cool for 5 to 10 minutes.

- A salmon filet is being baked on a sheet pan.

- Prepare the vegetables. While the salmon cools, heat 1 tablespoon olive oil in a large skillet and sauté the onion and bell pepper for 6 to 8 minutes, or until tender and translucent. Remove from the heat and set aside to cool.

- In a pan, veggies were cooked.

- Prepare the patties. Remove the skin from the cooled salmon and flake it into a large mixing basin with your hands. Combine the onion, bell pepper, dill, parsley, mayonnaise, Dijon mustard, garlic, almond flour, and eggs in a large mixing bowl. Mix all of the ingredients together with your hands until fully combined. Then, using your hands, shape the salmon mixture into small patties and set them aside. Pro Tip: To make it easier to transfer the formed patties to the burner, set them on a parchment-lined baking sheet.

- Salmon patties are being made.

- Make the patties. In a large skillet over medium heat, heat several teaspoons of olive oil and fry the salmon patties for 3 to 4 minutes on each side. Transfer the salmon patties to a plate lined with paper towels.

- In a pan, fish patties were cooked.

- Prepare the lemon-dill sauce. In a small mixing bowl, add the mayonnaise, chopped dill, lemon zest and juice, salt, and pepper.

- In a mixing bowl, combine the lemon dill sauce.

- Serve. With the lemon dill sauce, serve the salmon patties.

- Instead of pan frying, spray a baking sheet with oil spray (my favorite is avocado oil) and bake at 400°F for 10 to 12 minutes on each side.

- King Salmon has a high oil content and is a moister fish by nature. If using King Salmon, you may only need one beaten egg.

- Canned salmon is often dryer than fresh salmon. To keep your salmon patties moist, you may wish to double the mayonnaise to 1/4 cup.

- I've made a big batch of these for dinner prep, and they're fantastic. They freeze and reheat perfectly.

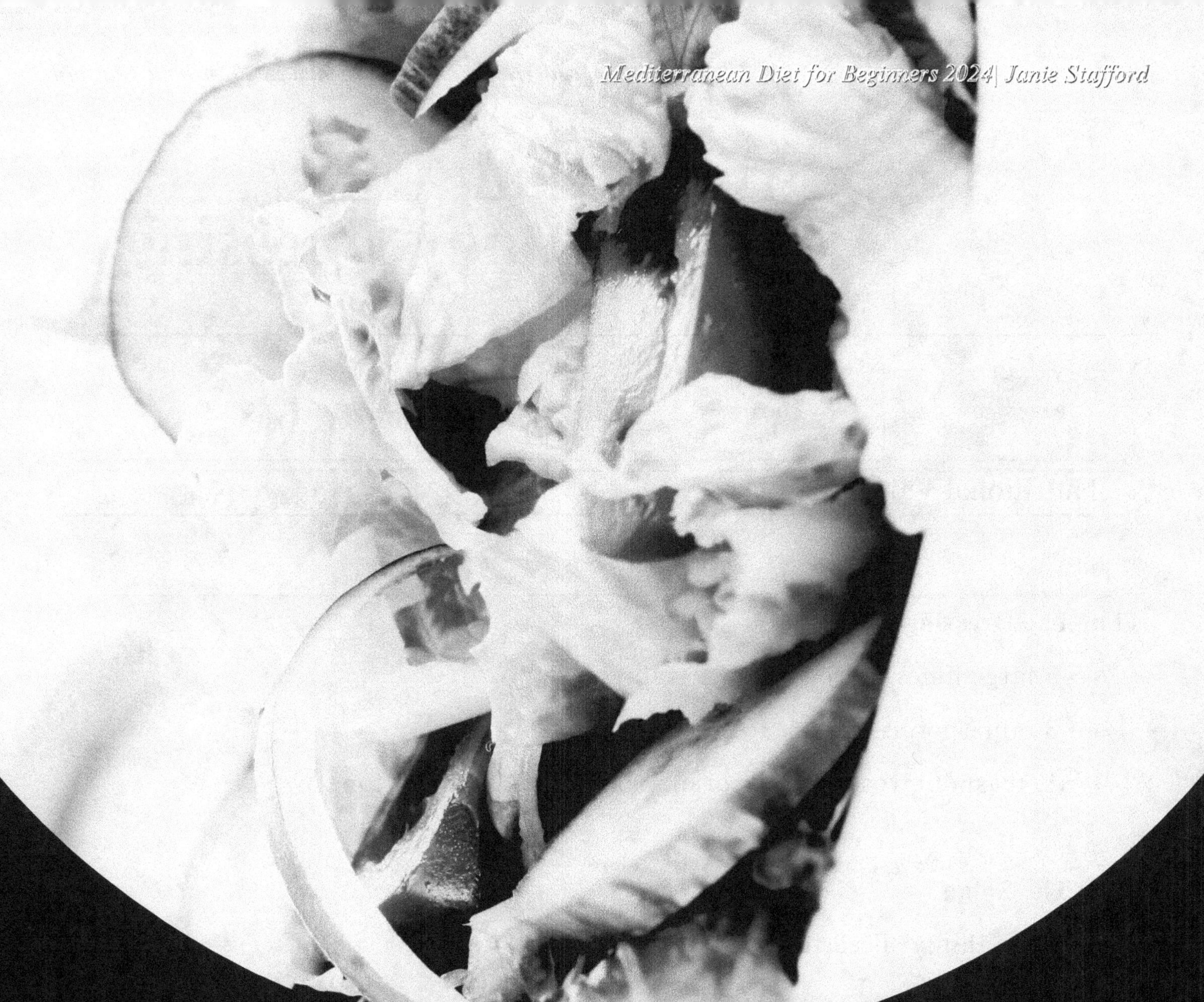

SIDES, SALADS AND SOUP

RECIPES

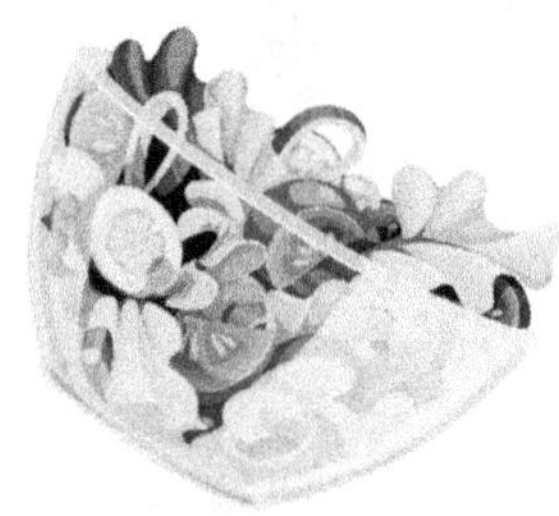

Fruit Salad with Citrus Honey Dressing

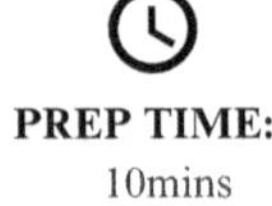			
PREP TIME: 10mins	**COOK TIME:** 15mins	**SERVINGS:** 6	**COURSE:** Appetizer

Nutritional Value:	Calories: 135.5kcal	Fat: 4.8g	Carb: 25.2g	Protein: 2.4g

INGREDIENTS:

For The Dressing

- • 3 large limes, juiced (about 6 tablespoons)
- • 3 tablespoons honey
- • ½ teaspoon rosewater or orange blossom water (optional)

For The Salad

- 2 cups thinly sliced fresh strawberries
- 1 cup fresh cherries, pitted and halved
- 1 cup blackberries
- ½ cup raspberries
- ¼ cup pomegranate seeds (optional)
- ⅓ cup roughly chopped walnuts, raw or toasted
- 2 tablespoons roughly chopped fresh mint leaves

DIRECTIONS:

- Prepare the dressing. Stir together the lime juice and honey in a small saucepan over medium heat. Stir for about 2 minutes, or until the honey is mixed and the mixture is warm. Remove from the heat and, if using, whisk in the rosewater. Place aside to cool.

- Combine the salad ingredients. Combine the strawberries, cherries, blackberries, raspberries, and pomegranate seeds (if using) in a large mixing basin. Add the dressing and gently mix the fruit to incorporate.

- Finish by serving. Gently stir in the walnuts and mint. Serve the salad on a plate or in individual bowls.

NOTES:

- Feel free to substitute any seasonal fruits you have on hand.

- This dish is adapted from my first cookbook, which is available almost anywhere books are sold.

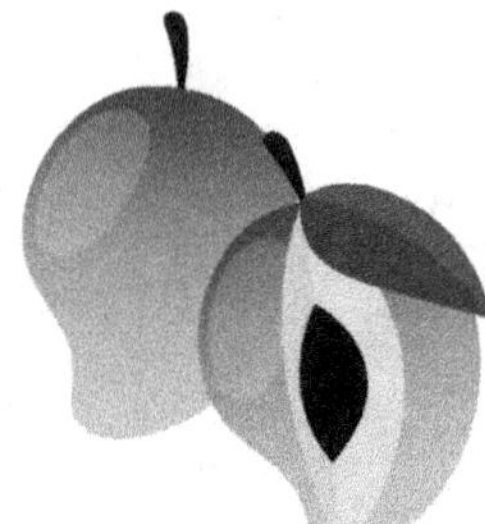

Grilled Mango with Lime, Aleppo Pepper, and Honey

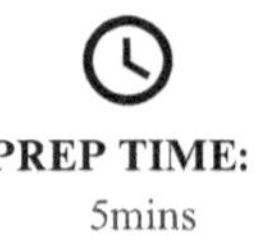

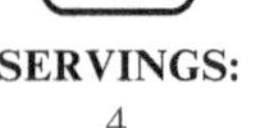
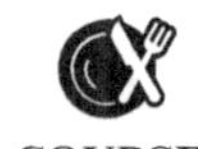

PREP TIME:	**COOK TIME:**	**SERVINGS:**	**COURSE:**
5mins	1min	4	Appetizer, Dessert or Side Dish

Nutritional Value:	Calories: 129.2kcal	Fat: 0.8g	Carb: 32.8g	Protein: 1.8g

INGREDIENTS:

- Extra virgin olive oil
- 4 ripe mangos
- 1 lime, halved
- Kosher salt
- Aleppo pepper or red chili flakes
- Warmed honey, for drizzling (optional)

DIRECTIONS:

- Prepare yourself: Heat the grill or a large indoor griddle pan to medium heat and lightly oil the grates.

- Slice the mango: Place a mango on its buttocks. Cut off one side with a sharp knife, slicing as close to the seed as possible. (Yes, mangos have seeds rather than pits!) Cut the mango in half lengthwise to produce two pieces. Continue with the remaining mangoes, discarding the seeds.

- Score the mango flesh in a grid or diamond pattern with a small knife, without cutting through the peel. Brush with olive oil lightly.

- Grill the mangos, flesh side down, on a hot grill. Grill for 1-2 minutes, or until charred. Take the pan off the heat and immediately squeeze the lime over the top. Season with kosher salt and Aleppo pepper (or red pepper flakes of choice).

- When the mangos are cool enough to handle, carefully push the skin back to release the mango flesh. Drizzle with warmed honey if desired. Serve hot.

NOTES:

- Select ripe but firm mangos. Mangoes that are ripe but not overly soft will maintain their shape better on the grill. Make sure the grill is hot: you want to rapidly obtain a good char and caramelization on the mango. This preserves some of the luscious raw flavor and texture

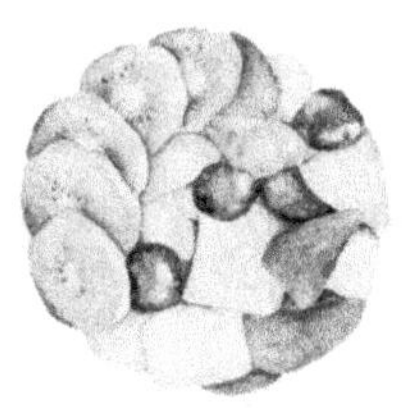

Winter Fruit Salad

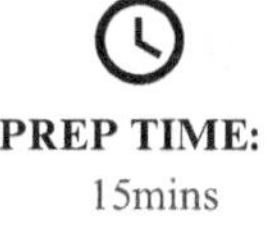			
PREP TIME: 15mins	**COOK TIME:** 0min	**SERVINGS:** 6	**COURSE:** Salad

Nutritional Value:	Calories: 230.7kcal	Fat: 7.2g	Carb: 43.9g	Protein: 3.3g

INGREDIENTS:

- For The Dressing:
- 2 to 3 tablespoons honey, warmed
- Juice of 2 large limes
- ¼ cup orange juice.

For The Salad:

- 2 large apples, cored and thinly sliced (Honeycrisp or gala apples will work)
- 2 Bosc pears, cored and thinly sliced
- 3 Clementine oranges, peeled and segmented
- 3 kiwis, peeled and thinly sliced into rounds
- 1 cup pomegranate arils
- ½ cup chopped walnuts
- 6 to 10 fresh mint leaves, chopped (optional)

DIRECTIONS:

- To make the dressing, follow these steps: Whisk together the dressing ingredients (honey, lime juice, and orange juice) in a large mixing basin.
- Add the fruit: Mix in all of the fruit and walnuts. If used, sprinkle with mint. Toss everything together until everything is fully integrated. Serve

NOTES:

- Sprinkle a couple tablespoons of unsweetened shredded coconut on top for more flavor and a Mediterranean flair.
- You might also try 1 tablespoon pomegranate molasses in the dressing. Pomegranate molasses is fantastic in salad dressings because it gives a unique bright tangy-sweet tone.

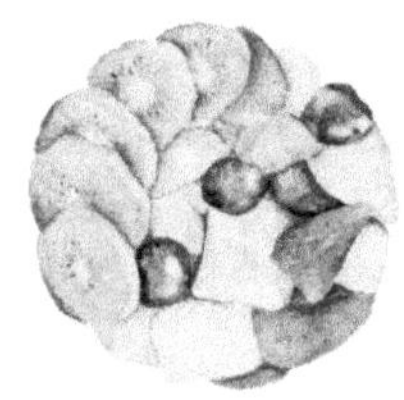

Easy Cucumber Salad

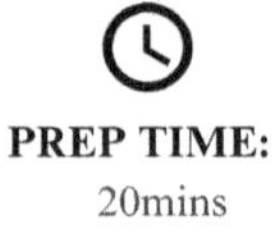 **PREP TIME:** 20mins	 **COOK TIME:** 0min	 **SERVINGS:** 4 servings	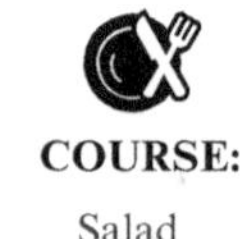 **COURSE:** Salad

Nutritional Value:	Calories: 37kcal	Fat: 0.3g	Carb: 8g	Protein: 1g

INGREDIENTS:

- 2 large English cucumbers, thinly sliced
- 1 tablespoon kosher salt
- ½ red onion, thinly sliced
- 2 green onions, thinly sliced
- 3 tablespoons fresh dill, chopped
- 1½ tablespoon champagne vinegar, or white wine vinegar
- 2 teaspoons honey
- freshly ground black pepper, to taste

DIRECTIONS:

- Cucumbers should be salted. Toss the cucumber slices in a colander with the salt.
- Salting cucumbers for cucumber salad
- Cucumbers should be washed and drained. As the salt draws moisture from the cucumbers, place the colander in the sink or on top of a dish. Allow this to sit for 20 minutes before rinsing the cucumber with cool water.
- Cucumber salad requires rinsing with water.
- In a mixing dish, combine the salad ingredients. Combine the drained cucumber, red onion, green onion, and fresh dill in a salad bowl.
- In a large mixing basin, combine the cucumber salad ingredients
- Prepare the dressing. In a second small bowl, combine the vinegar and honey, then drizzle over the salad.
- Dressing for cucumber salad in a small basin with a spoon.
- Garnish with black pepper and fresh dill leaves if desired.

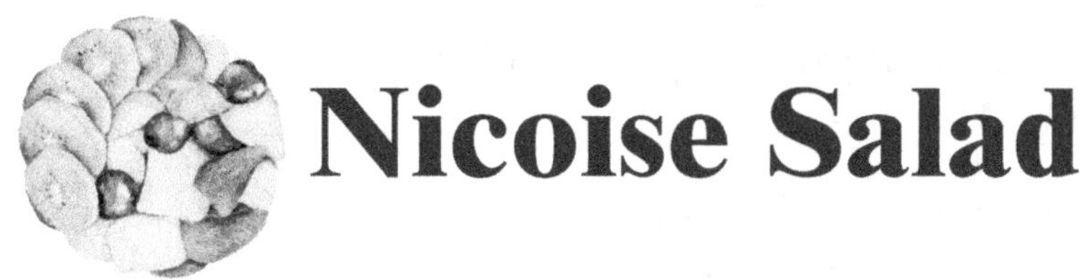

Nicoise Salad

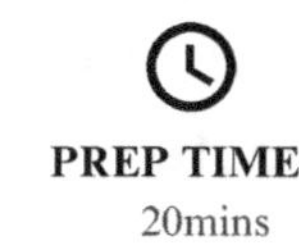			
PREP TIME: 20mins	**COOK TIME:** 25mins	**SERVINGS:** 6 servings	**COURSE:** Salad

Nutritional Value:	Calories: 247kcal	Fat: 18g	Carb: 16g	Protein: 6g

INGREDIENTS:

NICOISE SALAD

- 4 cups mixed salad greens
- 6 ounces green beans (haricot verts)
- 4 large eggs
- 2 cups baby red or white potatoes
- 1 (5-ounce) can tuna, drained
- 1 cup pitted olives
- 1 cup grape tomatoes, halved
- ½ English Cucumber, thinly sliced
- ½ small red onion, thinly sliced

LEMON VINAIGRETTE

- ⅓ cup extra virgin olive oil
- ¼ cup lemon juice
- 1 teaspoon Dijon mustard
- ½ teaspoon honey
- 1 garlic clove, minced
- kosher salt and freshly ground black pepper, to taste

DIRECTIONS:

- Making the vinaigrette. In a small bowl, whisk together all of the ingredients. Place aside.

- Salad dressing from Nicoise

- Bring the eggs to a boil. A small saucepan of water should be brought to a boil. Then, remove from the heat (so there are no bubbles) and gently fold in the eggs. Return the eggs to the pan and cook for 612 to 7 minutes for a somewhat jammy yolk. Cook for another 3 to 4 minutes if you prefer hard-boiled eggs.

- In a pot, boil eggs for Nicoise salad.

- The eggs should be chilled. Transfer the eggs to an ice water bath for a few minutes using a slotted spoon or skimmer. Then, crack, peel, and cut each one in half

- Prepare the potatoes. While the eggs are cooking, heat a medium saucepan of salted water to a boil. Reduce the heat to a simmer and boil the potatoes until cooked, about 15 minutes. Remove the potatoes with a slotted spoon (leaving the boiling water in the saucepan), transfer to a chopping board, and set aside to cool. Then cut in half.

- Boil the beans. Add the green beans to the pot and cook for 1 to 2 minutes, or until brilliant green. The beans should then be chilled in an ice water bath before draining in a colander.

- Make the Nicoise salad. Arrange the salad greens on a big plate. On top, layer the potatoes, green beans, tuna, tomatoes, olives, red onion, and soft-boiled eggs. Season with freshly ground black pepper and kosher salt. Drizzle the salad with the lemon vinaigrette. I use about half of the vinaigrette and keep the rest in the fridge for later use.

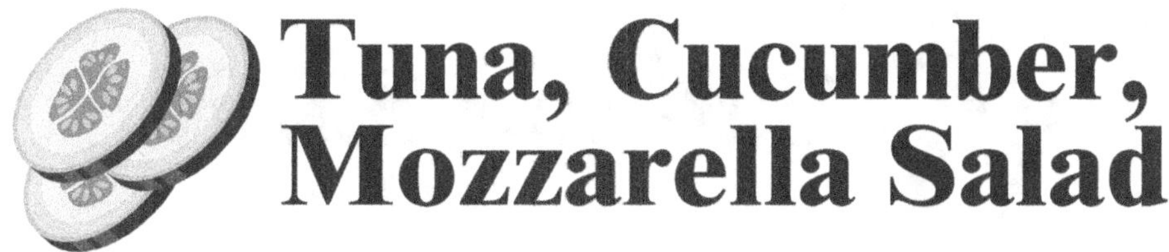

Tuna, Cucumber, Mozzarella Salad

	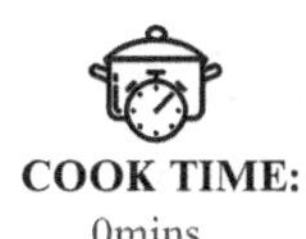		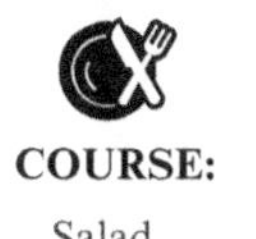
PREP TIME: 10mins	**COOK TIME:** 0mins	**SERVINGS:** 4 servings	**COURSE:** Salad

Nutritional Value:	Calories: 144kcal	Fat: 7g	Carb: 9g	Protein: 14g

INGREDIENTS:

- 4 cups lettuce spring mix
- 1 (5-ounce) can tuna, drained
- 4 Bocconcini mozzarella balls
- ½ English Cucumber
- 1 small shallot
- ⅔ cup sweet corn, cooked and chilled
- ½ recipe lemon vinaigrette

DIRECTIONS:

- Slice. Slice the mozzarella balls, cucumber, and shallot thinly
- Cucumber, shallot, and mozzarella slicing for tuna salad
- Toss. Toss the lettuce with the tuna, mozzarella, cucumber, shallot, and corn in a large mixing basin. Drizzle with the lemon vinaigrette and mix well.

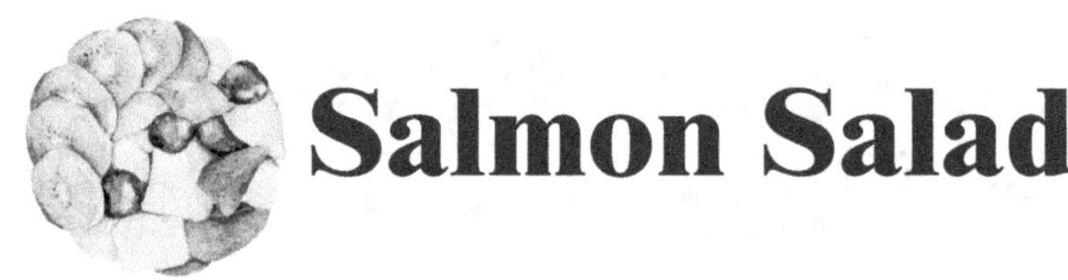

Salmon Salad

 **PREP TIME:** 15mins	 **COOK TIME:** 20mins	 **SERVINGS:** 4 servings	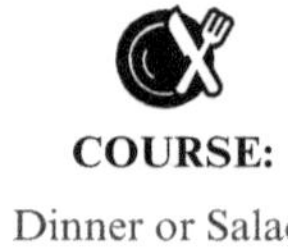 **COURSE:** Dinner or Salad

Nutritional Value:	Calories: 361kcal	Fat: 25g	Carb: 4g	Protein: 29g

INGREDIENTS:

- **FOR THE SALMON**
- 1 ¼ pounds salmon filet
- ½ tablespoon olive oil
- 1 teaspoon smoked paprika
- kosher salt and freshly ground black pepper, to taste
- **FOR THE DRESSING**
- ⅓ cup mayonnaise
- ½ lemon, zested and juiced (about ½ tablespoon of zest and 1 ½ tablespoons juice)
- 2 teaspoons Dijon mustard
- 1 garlic clove, minced
- kosher salt and freshly ground black pepper, to taste
- **FOR THE SALAD**
- ½ small red onion, finely diced
- 3 large radishes, grated
- 2 stalks celery, small diced
- 2 tablespoons finely chopped fresh dill
- 2 tablespoons finely chopped fresh chives

DIRECTIONS:

- Make the salmon. Preheat the oven to 375 degrees Fahrenheit (190 degrees Celsius). Place the fish on a baking sheet lined with parchment paper. Drizzle olive oil over the salmon and season with smoked paprika, salt, and pepper.

- Bake the fish and flake it. Bake for 16–18 minutes (depending on size and thickness), or until the salmon flakes easily with a fork. Allow it to cool to room temperature before flaking the salmon into chunks and placing it in a bowl. Refrigerate the flakes salmon for 5 to 10 minutes.

- Cut the vegetables into dice. Add the onion, radish, celery, dill, and chives to the flakes salmon.

- Prepare the dressing. Make the dressing in a separate small bowl. Combine the mayonnaise, lemon zest and juice, mustard, garlic, salt, and pepper in a mixing bowl.

- Creamy salmon salad dressing in a bowl

- Mix everything together. Pour the dressing over the salad and toss lightly to mix.

- In a bowl, creamy salmon salad

- Serve the salmon salad cold, either on butter lettuce leaves or as a sandwich or wrap.

NOTES:

- The salmon can be baked in a baking dish or on a conventional half sheet pan, but I like quarter sheet pans. They're the ideal size for baking full filets of fish!

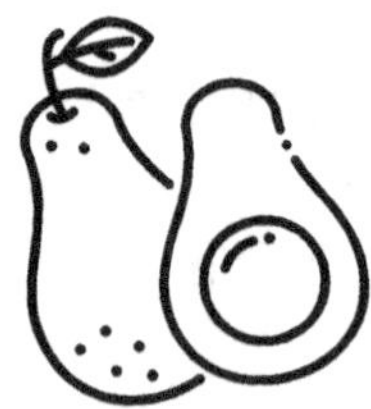

Salmon Avocado Salad

 **PREP TIME:** 10mins	 **COOK TIME:** 10mins	 **SERVINGS:** 2 servings	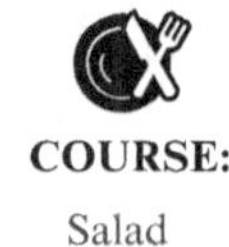 **COURSE:** Salad

Nutritional Value:	Calories: 732kcal	Fat: 56g	Carb: 21g	Protein: 40g

INGREDIENTS:

SALMON AVOCADO SALAD

- 4 cups baby spinach
- 2 tomatoes, chopped
- 1 avocado, diced
- 1 cucumber, peeled and sliced
- 1/4 cup red onion, chopped

- 2 tablespoon olive oil
- 2 salmon filets
- salt and pepper, to taste

DRESSING

- 1 recipe lemon vinaigrette

DIRECTIONS:

- In a large skillet over medium-high heat, heat the olive oil. Season both sides of the salmon filets with salt and pepper. Cook the salmon filets, top side down, for 4-5 minutes.

- Cook for a further 2-3 minutes, or until the salmon is mostly opaque with just a hint of softness in the center.

- Divide the remaining salad ingredients between two bowls, then top with the cooked salmon.

- In a small dish, combine the dressing ingredients and drizzle on top.

NOTES:

- The remaining dressing can be used on future salads or as a marinade for meat. It's also delicious on chicken!

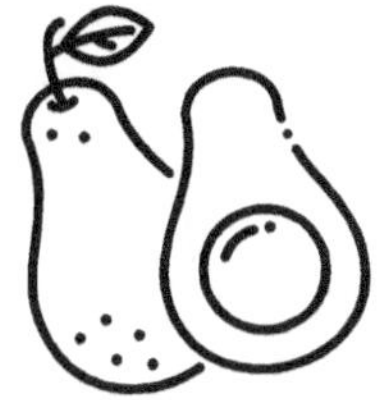

Tomato Avocado Salad

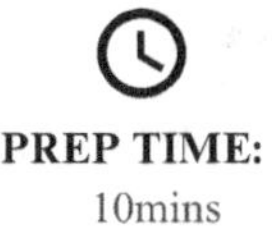	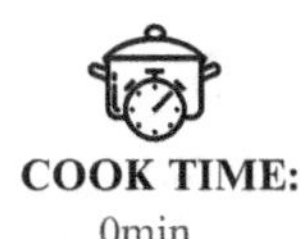		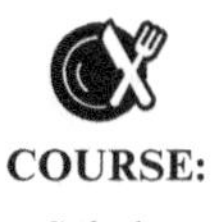
PREP TIME: 10mins	**COOK TIME:** 0min	**SERVINGS:** 4 servings	**COURSE:** Salad

Nutritional Value:	Calories: 171kcal	Fat: 15g	Carb: 11g	Protein: 2g

INGREDIENTS:

- 4 vine-ripened tomatoes, thinly sliced
- ¼ onion, thinly sliced
- 1 small avocado, thinly sliced
- 1 tablespoon finely chopped parsley
- 2 tablespoon extra-virgin olive oil
- ½ lemon, juiced (about 1 ½ tablespoons)
- kosher salt and freshly ground black pepper, to taste

DIRECTIONS:

- On a big plate or serving tray, arrange the thinly sliced tomatoes.
- A serving of sliced tomatoes for avocado salad
- On top, arrange the sliced onions.
- For an avocado salad, a platter of sliced tomatoes and onion
- Then add the avocado slices and parsley
- Salad of tomato, onion, and avocado
- Before serving, drizzle with lemon juice and olive oil and season with salt and pepper.

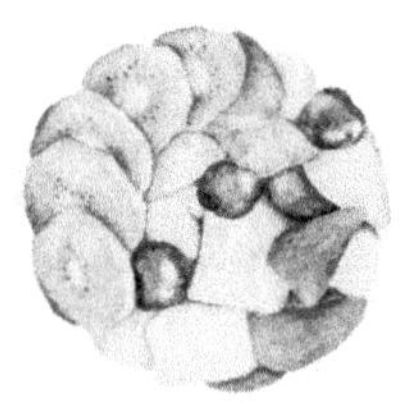

Israeli Salad

PREP TIME:	COOK TIME:	SERVINGS:	COURSE:
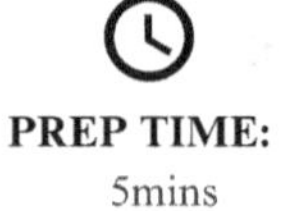			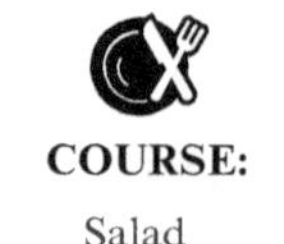
5mins	0min	4 servings	Salad

Nutritional Value:	Calories: 79kcal	Fat: 4g	Carb: 10g	Protein: 2g

INGREDIENTS:

- 2 cups diced tomatoes
- 2 cups diced cucumber
- 1 cup orange bell pepper, or any color
- 1/4 cup diced red onion
- 1/3 cup finely chopped flat-leaf parsley
- 2 tbsp finely chopped mint
- 2 tbsp fresh lemon juice
- 1 tbsp olive oil
- salt and pepper, to taste

DIRECTIONS:

- Stir together all of the ingredients in a mixing basin.
- Serve immediately or store in the refrigerator for up to 2 days.

VEGETABLE MAINS AND MEATLESS

RECIPES

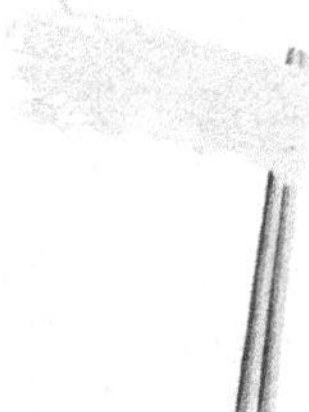

Zucchini Noodle Caprese

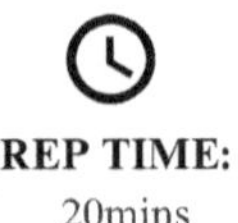 **PREP TIME:** 20mins	 **COOK TIME:** 0min	 **SERVINGS:** 5 Servings	 **COURSE:** Main Course

Nutritional Value:	Calories: 352kcal	Fat: 30g	Carb: 10g	Protein: 12g

INGREDIENTS:

- 4 medium zucchini
- 8 ounces cherry tomatoes
- 8 ounces small balls of buffalo mozzarella, in water

BASIL PESTO

- 2 tbsp raw pine nuts, plus extra for garnish
- 1/4 cup raw cashews
- 1 cup packed basil leaves
- 1/3 cup olive oil
- 2 garlic cloves
- 1 tsp lemon juice
- 1/4 tsp salt
- black pepper, to taste

GARNISH

- toasted pine nuts
- fresh basil leaves

DIRECTIONS:

- Toss the pine nuts gently in a pan over medium-low heat for 5 minutes. Then put them in the food processor.

- Toss the cashews gently in the same skillet for 10 minutes. Then place it in your food processor.

- Except for the olive oil, combine the remaining pesto ingredients in a food processor. Pulse until all of the ingredients are combined. While carefully adding the olive oil into your food processor, turn it on. Set aside once your pesto has reached a smooth and creamy consistency.

- Remove the ends of each zucchini and spiralize to make zucchini noodles. Put these in a large mixing bowl.

- Cut the tomatoes in half and combine them with the zucchini in a mixing dish. Place your mozzarella balls in the same bowl after cutting them in half.

- Remove all of the pesto from the food processor and add it to the bowl with a spoon or spatula. Combine all of the ingredients until fully blended. Serve right away

NOTES:

- Because zucchini noodles absorb water over time, if you make this salad ahead of time, you may notice some liquid collecting at the bottom of your dish. To drain any surplus water, simply place the bowl over the sink.

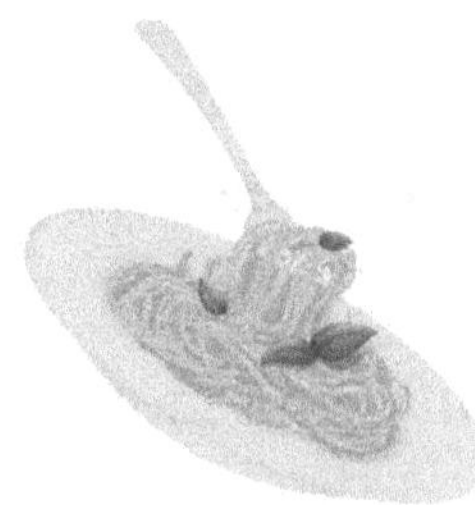

Spaghetti Squash, Brussels Sprouts, and Crispy Shallots

 **PREP TIME:** 15mins	 **COOK TIME:** 45mins	 **SERVINGS:** 4 Servings	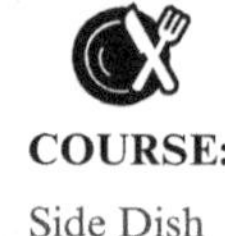 **COURSE:** Side Dish

Nutritional Value:	Calories: 154kcal	Fat: 11g	Carb: 13g	Protein: 4g

INGREDIENTS:

- 3 and a half to 4 pound spaghetti squash
- 3 tablespoons olive oil (divided)
- 2 large shallots, thinly sliced
- 1 pound Brussels sprouts, shaved or thinly sliced
- 3 garlic cloves, minced
- salt and pepper, to taste

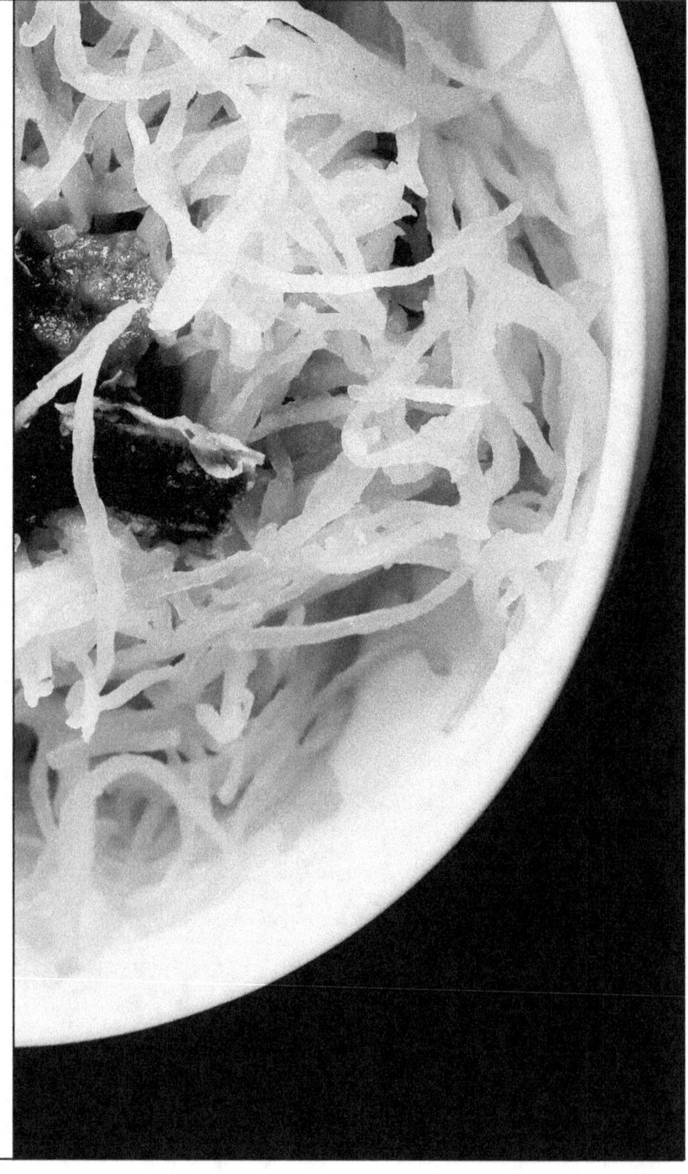

DIRECTIONS:

- Preheat the oven to 400 degrees Fahrenheit/200 degrees Celsius. Cut the spaghetti squash in half and remove the seeds. Coat the inside with olive oil, salt, and pepper, and bake for 40-50 minutes.

- For a side dish, spaghetti squash is seasoned and oiled.

- When the spaghetti squash has been cooking for about 30 minutes, heat 2 tablespoons olive oil in a big pan over medium heat. Cook, stirring regularly, for about 8 minutes, or until the shallots are gently brown and crispy.

- In a pan, crisp shallots are being sautéed.

- Remove the crispy shallots with a slotted spoon to a paper towel to drain.

- Brussels sprouts with crispy shallots in a pan

- Sauté the brussels sprouts and garlic in the same pan for 4-5 minutes. You may also need to add another splash of oil.

- When the spaghetti squash is done, take it from the oven and scrape the flesh into a bowl using a fork. Season with salt and pepper after adding the sautéed Brussels sprouts and crispy shallots to the bowl.

- In a large mixing dish, combine spaghetti squash, Brussels sprouts, and crispy shallots.

- Combine all of the ingredients and serve!

NOTES:

- To store: This can be stored in an airtight container in the fridge for up to 4 days.

- To reheat: Simply pop this in the microwave for about 1 minute or so.

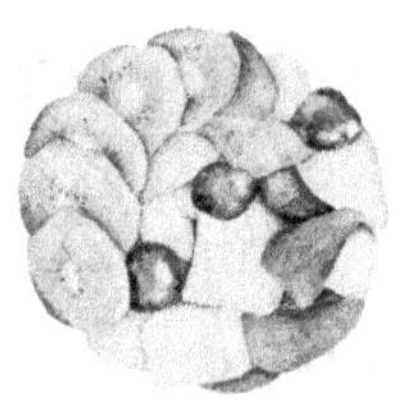

Sauteed Cabbage

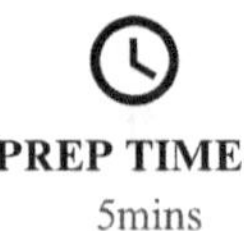 **PREP TIME:** 5mins	 **COOK TIME:** 15mins	 **SERVINGS:** 6 servings	 **COURSE:** Side Dish

Nutritional Value:	Calories: 80kcal	Fat: 5g	Carb: 9g	Protein: 2g

INGREDIENTS:

- 1 small head green cabbage, thinly sliced
- 1 onion, sliced
- 2 garlic cloves, minced
- 2 tablespoon ghee, or a blend of butter and olive oil
- salt and pepper, to taste

DIRECTIONS:

- Cut the cabbage in half, remove the core, and thinly slice it. The onions should next be cut into pieces.

- In a large skillet over medium-high heat, melt the ghee. Cook for a minute, or until the onions begin to soften. Then add the minced garlic and stir once more.

- Add the cabbage and cook for 12-15 minutes. During this time, stir the cabbage occasionally until it softens and caramelizes.

- Season with salt and pepper and stir to blend before serving.

NOTES:

- Because the cabbage may take up the majority of the pan, it's best to stir it using tongs. If your pan isn't large enough, sauté the cabbage in batches. However, cabbage, like spinach, will wilt once cooked.

Warm Sweet Potato Noodles, Cabbage, and Lentil Salad

**PREP TIME:** 15mins	**COOK TIME:** 20mins	**SERVINGS:** 4 Servings	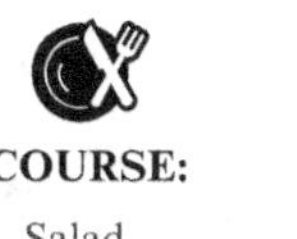**COURSE:** Salad

Nutritional Value:	Calories: 414.5kcal	Fat: 23g	Carb: 41.3g	Protein: 14.8g

INGREDIENTS:

- 1/2 cup green lentils
- 4 cups water
- 1 bay leaf
- 1 piece kombu seaweed, approx 4 inches long
- 1 sweet potato, spiralized
- 2 tbsp olive oil
- 1/2 yellow onion, sliced
- 4 leaves Swiss chard, sliced
- 2 cups sliced red cabbage
- 1/3 cup pine nuts, toasted
- 1 bunch parsley or cilantro
- 1 recipe Dijon Vinaigrette

DIRECTIONS:

- Fill a fine mesh sieve halfway with lentils. Examine and remove any undesirables before rinsing under the faucet.

- In a small pot, combine the lentils, water, bay leaf, and kombu. The lentils should be covered by about 2 inches of water. Bring the lentils to a boil, then reduce to a low heat, cover, and simmer for 20 minutes. The water should be at a low simmer with few bubbles.

- After the lentils have cooked for about 5 minutes, heat the olive oil and onion in a big pan over medium heat. Cook for 2-3 minutes, or until the onions are transparent. You can also sauté them till totally caramelized.

- Sauté the sliced Swiss chard in the pan for a minute. Then add the spiralized sweet potato and cook for 3 minutes, turning with tongs. Finally, add the sliced red cabbage to the skillet and cook for one minute, turning and stirring constantly. The salad should now be transferred to a large serving bowl.

- The lentils should be almost done at this point. Drain and rinse them before adding them to the salad.

- Toasted pine nuts, fresh herbs, and Dijon vinaigrette should be sprinkled over the salad. Toss all of the ingredients together and serve warm

NOTES:

- Sweet potato noodles that have been spiralized can be rather lengthy. Trim them using kitchen scissors before cooking to make them simpler to eat.

- Cooking the lentils with kombu seaweed not only gives a fantastic umami flavor, but it also improves digestibility by lowering phytic acid in the lentils.

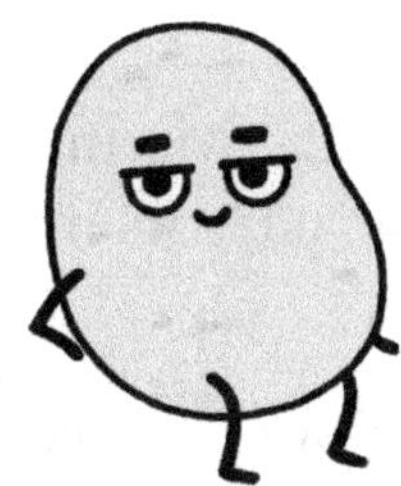

Sweet Potato Soup

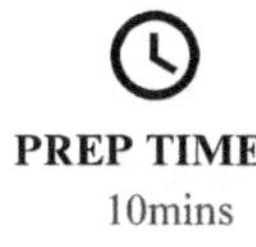			
PREP TIME: 10mins	**COOK TIME:** 30mins	**SERVINGS:** 4 People	**COURSE:** Soup

Nutritional Value:	Calories: 254kcal	Fat: 7g	Carb: 45g	Protein: 4g

INGREDIENTS:

- 2 tablespoons avocado oil, or olive oil
- 3 carrots, sliced
- 1 yellow onion
- 1 1/2 pound sweet potatoes, peeled and diced
- 2 garlic cloves, minced
- 1 tablespoon fresh ginger, finely chopped
- 1/4 teaspoon red pepper flakes
- 1/4 teaspoon paprika
- 4 cups vegetable broth, or more for thinner consistency

GARNISH

- watercress
- pistachios
- coconut cream or yogurt
- red pepper flakes
- cracked black pepper

DIRECTIONS:

- In a large stockpot over medium high heat, heat the oil. Stir in the diced onion and carrots for 6-8 minutes, or until the carrots have softened somewhat.

- Combine the garlic, ginger, red pepper flakes, and paprika in a mixing bowl. Stir for 2-3 minutes, or until the mixture is aromatic.

- Add the sweet potato dices and veggie broth. Bring the water to a boil over high heat. Reduce the heat to low, cover, and leave to cook for 15-20 minutes, or until the sweet potato is fork tender

- Transfer the soup ingredients to a high-powered blender using a ladle. Blend for one minute on high, or until creamy. For a thinner consistency, add extra broth or water.

- Pour into a serving dish and top with coconut cream or yogurt, chopped pistachios, red pepper flakes, crushed black pepper, and watercress.

NOTES:

- If you use more than 1 1/2 pounds of sweet potato, you may surpass the maximum fill line on your blender.

- Remember that you may always add a little water or broth to thin it down if necessary.

CELERY ROOT PUREE WITH BALSAMIC ROASTED BEETS AND PEARL ONIONS

 **PREP TIME:** 20mins	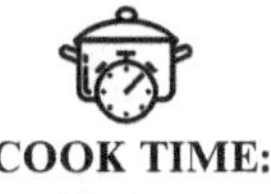 **COOK TIME:** 45mins	 **SERVINGS:** 4	 **COURSE:** Main Course or Side Dish

Nutritional Value:	Calories: 441kcal	Fat: 20g	Carb: 30g	Protein: 6g

INGREDIENTS:

- **BALSAMIC ROASTED BEETS AND PEARL ONIONS**
- 4 beets
- 1 1/2 cups pearl onions
- 3 tbsp olive oil, (divided)
- salt and pepper, to taste
- 2 tbsp balsamic vinegar
- 1/2 tbsp maple syrup
- 1 tbsp fresh thyme leaves
- 1 tbsp fresh tarragon, chopped
- **CELERY ROOT PUREE**
- 1 tbsp olive oil
- 3 cloves garlic, finely chopped
- 4 cups celery root, peeled and diced into 1/2 inch cubes
- 13.5 oz full-fat coconut milk
- 2/3 cup water
- salt and pepper, to taste
- **TOPPING**
- 2 cups microgreens

DIRECTIONS:

- Preheat the oven to 400 degrees F.

- Drain and rinse pearl onions if using a jar or can. If using fresh pearl onions, soak them for 5 minutes in a bowl of warm water to soften the skin. Remove the outer skin and snip off the ends with a pairing knife. Place the chicken on a large baking pan and set aside.

- Peel the beets with a vegetable peeler and set on a non-wood cutting board (a wood cutting board will stain). Place the beets on a baking sheet in quarters or uniformly sized slices. Season with salt and pepper and toss with 2 tablespoons olive oil. Cook for 25-30 minutes, stirring once or twice halfway through, in the center of the oven.

- Combine the balsamic vinegar, maple syrup, herbs, and 1 tablespoon olive oil in a mixing bowl. Place aside.

- While the beets cook, heat the olive oil in a saucepan over medium-high heat and sauté the garlic for one minute. Add the celery root, coconut milk, water, salt, and pepper to taste. Bring the liquid to a boil, then reduce to a low heat, cover, and leave to simmer for 15 minutes.

- Turn off the heat and purée the celery root mixture with a stick blender until smooth. Cover and keep warm until ready to serve. (*Alternatively, purée the ingredients in a high-powered blender).

- After the beets and onions have finished cooking, drizzle the balsamic mixture over them, toss to incorporate, and simmer for another 5 minutes.

- To serve, spoon some celery root puree into a bowl and top with roasted beets, pearl onions, and a handful of microgreens.

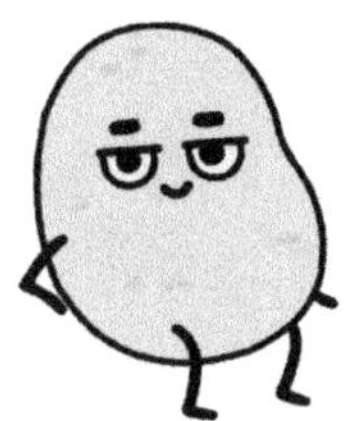

Baked Sweet Potato

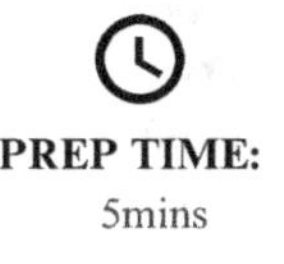 **PREP TIME:** 5mins	 **COOK TIME:** 1hr	 **SERVINGS:** 4 Servings	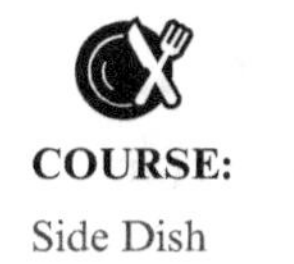 **COURSE:** Side Dish

Nutritional Value:	Calories: 102kcal	Fat: 0.2g	Carb: 23.6g	Protein: 2.3g

INGREDIENTS:

- 4 sweet potatoes
- kosher salt and freshly ground black pepper, to taste
- butter, optional

DIRECTIONS:

- Preheat the oven to 400 degrees Fahrenheit (200 degrees Celsius). Scrub and wash your sweet potatoes thoroughly.

- The sweet potato is being washed under the faucet.

- Place the sweet potatoes on a baking sheet and use a fork or sharp knife to poke 4 to 5 holes in each sweet potato.

- Using a fork, poke the sweet potato.

- Bake for 60 minutes, or until the potatoes are tender. Poke them with a fork or knife to see whether they're done. When inserted, there should be very little resistance.

NOTES:

- If you don't have a good baking sheet, I highly recommend purchasing a heavy duty baking sheet that won't warp or twist in the oven.

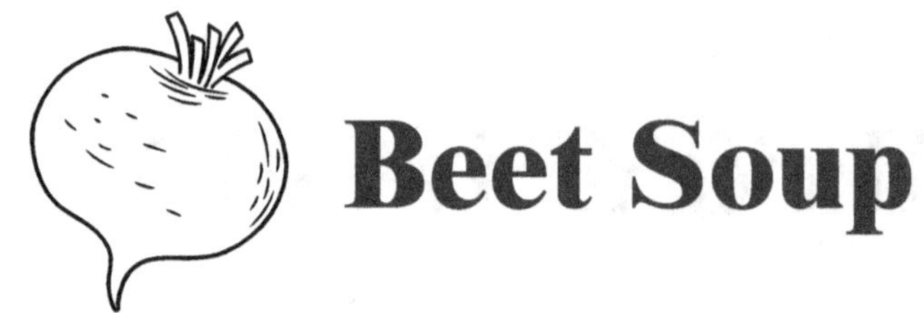

Beet Soup

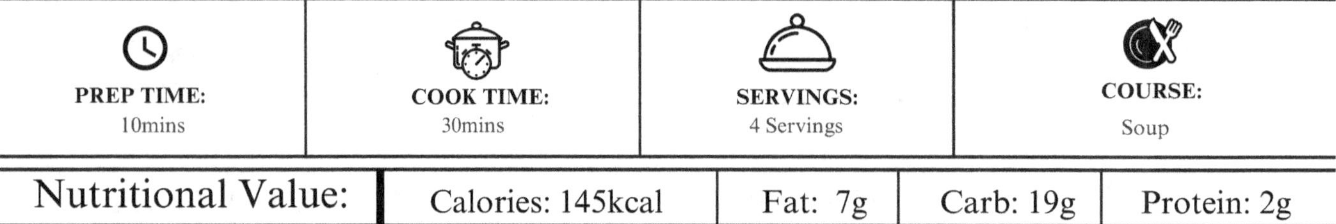

PREP TIME: 10mins	**COOK TIME:** 30mins	**SERVINGS:** 4 Servings	**COURSE:** Soup

Nutritional Value:	Calories: 145kcal	Fat: 7g	Carb: 19g	Protein: 2g

INGREDIENTS:

- 2 tablespoons avocado oil, or olive oil
- 1 yellow onion
- 3 garlic cloves, minced
- 1 tablespoon fresh ginger, peeled and finely chopped
- salt and pepper, to taste
- 3 large beets, peeled and diced (or 4 beets, if smaller)
- 1 medium parsnip, peeled and diced (approx 1 cup)
- 4 cups vegetable broth, or more for desired texture

GARNISH

- coconut cream or yogurt
- parsley
- black sesame seeds
- cracked black pepper

DIRECTIONS:

- In a large stockpot over medium high heat, heat the avocado oil. Cook for 3-4 minutes, or until the onion has softened.

- Cook for an additional 1-2 minutes, until the garlic, ginger, salt, and pepper are aromatic.

- Combine the chopped beets, diced parsnips, and vegetable broth in a mixing bowl. Bring the water to a boil over high heat. Reduce the heat to low, cover the saucepan, and cook for 25-30 minutes, or until the beets are tender with a fork.

- Transfer the soup to a high-powered blender using a ladle. Blend for one minute, or until the mixture is creamy.

- Pour the soup into a bowl and top with coconut cream or yogurt, parsley, black sesame seeds, and crushed black pepper to serve.

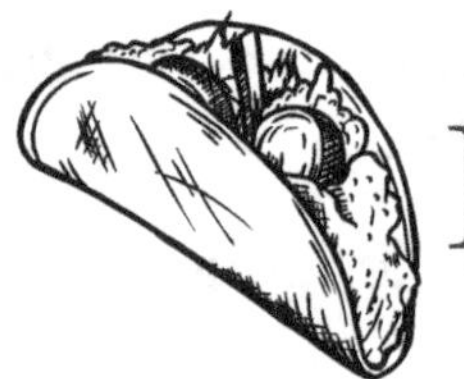

Easy Veggie Wrap

PREP TIME:	**COOK TIME:**	**SERVINGS:**	**COURSE:**
30mins	0min	4	Main Course

Nutritional Value:	Calories: 347kcal	Fat: 8g	Carb: 55g	Protein: 12g

INGREDIENTS:

- 1 medium cucumber
- ½ teaspoon (plus a couple pinches) of salt divided
- 1 medium tomato diced
- ¼ red onion diced
- ¼ green pepper diced
- 4 tablespoons chopped kalamata olives
- 1 jar (540 grams / 19 oz) chickpeas
- 200 grams (7 oz) vegan yogurt (I used soy)
- 2 tablespoons chopped fresh dill
- 1 clove of garlic minced
- 1 tablespoon lemon juice
- Pepper to taste
- 2 cups (112 grams) chopped lettuce
- 4 large tortillas

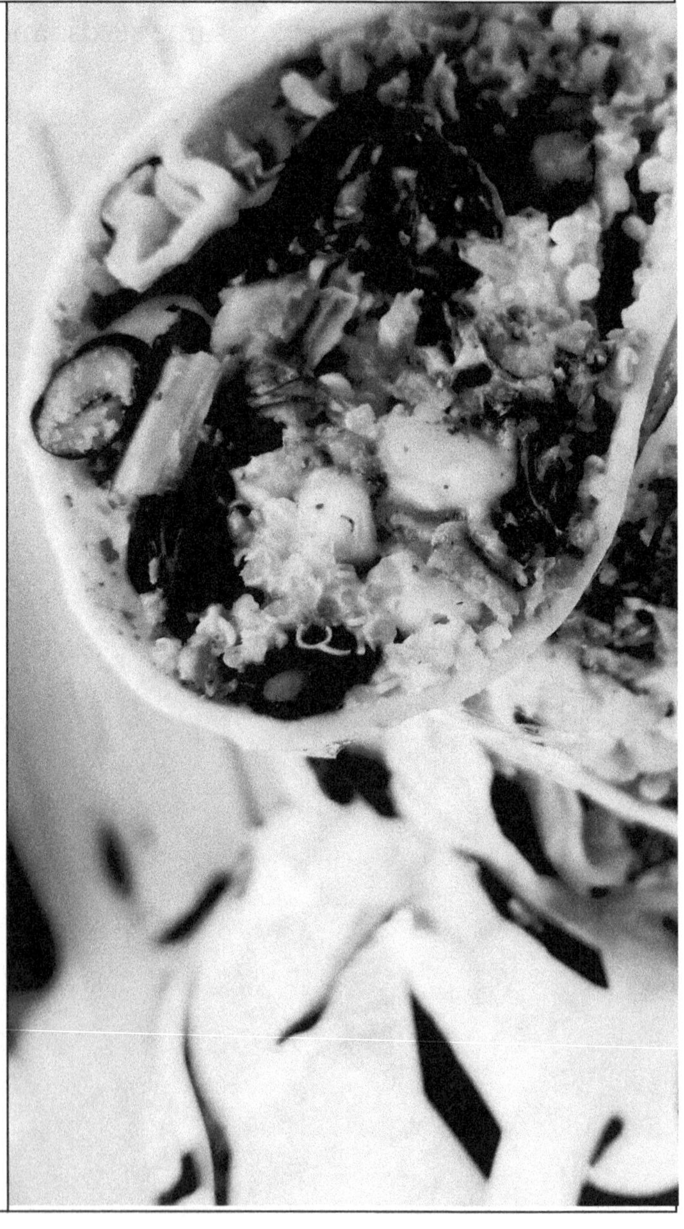

DIRECTIONS:

- Grate half of the cucumber and season with salt to taste. Place it in a sieve over a bowl and set
aside to drain while you chop the rest of your vegetables. Dice the other half of the cucumber as well. Combine the cucumber, tomato, red onion, green pepper, and black olives in a mixing
bowl.

- Place the chickpeas in a bowl after draining and rinsing them. Use your hands or a fork to crush them

- Squeeze as much water as possible from the shredded cucumber. Combine the grated cucumber, vegan yogurt, dill, garlic, lemon juice, and a pinch of salt and pepper in a mixing bowl.

- To the mashed chickpeas, add 3 tablespoons tzatziki and 12 teaspoon salt and pepper. Combine thoroughly.

- Make the wraps with a handful of lettuce, smashed chickpeas, diced vegetables, and tzatziki. If desired, toast the finished wraps in a dry skillet over medium-high heat. Begin with the seam side down to prevent them from unraveling.

Garlicky Spinach and Chickpea Soup with Lemon and Pecorino Romano

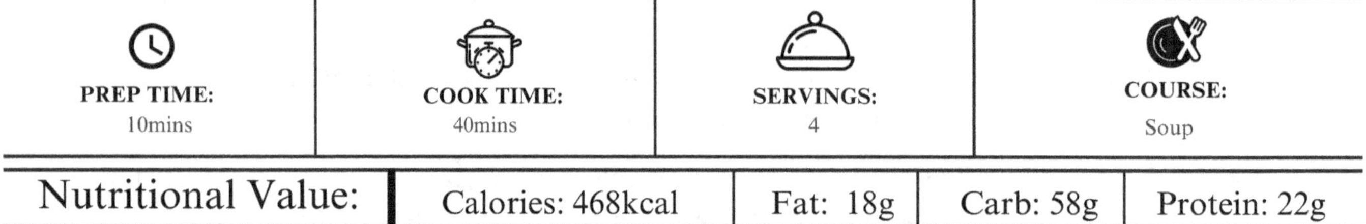

PREP TIME:	COOK TIME:	SERVINGS:	COURSE:
10mins	40mins	4	Soup

Nutritional Value:	Calories: 468kcal	Fat: 18g	Carb: 58g	Protein: 22g

INGREDIENTS:

- Two 15-ounce cans chickpeas

- Extra-virgin olive oil

- 1 large yellow onion, roughly chopped

- 4 or 5 large garlic cloves, minced

- Kosher salt

- 1 teaspoon ground cumin

- 1 teaspoon ground coriander

- ¾ teaspoon sweet paprika

- ½ teaspoon crushed red pepper flakes

- ½ teaspoon freshly ground black pepper

- 4 cups vegetable stock or low-sodium chicken broth

- 2 cups (packed) fresh baby spinach (2 to 3 ounces)

- ½ cup roughly chopped fresh flat-leaf parsley

- 1 large lemon, cut in half

- ½ cup grated Pecorino Romano cheese

- Crusty bread, for serving

DIRECTIONS:

- Drain the chickpeas, reserving 12 cup liquid.

- Heat 3 tablespoons olive oil in a large pot over medium heat until shimmering. Season with a generous amount of salt (approximately 12 tsp) and the onion and garlic. Cook, stirring frequently, over medium heat until aromatic, about 5 minutes. Cook, stirring frequently, for about 30 seconds, after adding the cumin, coriander, paprika, red pepper flakes, and black pepper.

- Stir in the chickpeas to coat with the spices. Mash the chickpeas coarsely using a potato masher or the back of a sturdy fork (you're just wanting to break some of them up).

- Combine the stock and the saved chickpea liquid in a mixing bowl. Increase the heat to high and bring to a boil for 5 minutes. Reduce the heat to medium-low and cover the pot partially with the lid. Cook for 30 minutes with the chickpeas.

- Turn off the heat. Allow the soup to settle for 1 minute, or until the spinach wilts, after adding the spinach and parsley. Squeeze half a lemon over the soup, stir, and season with extra lemon juice to taste.

- Transfer the soup to serving bowls and garnish with a splash of olive oil and some shredded Pecorino Romano cheese. With crusty bread, serve.

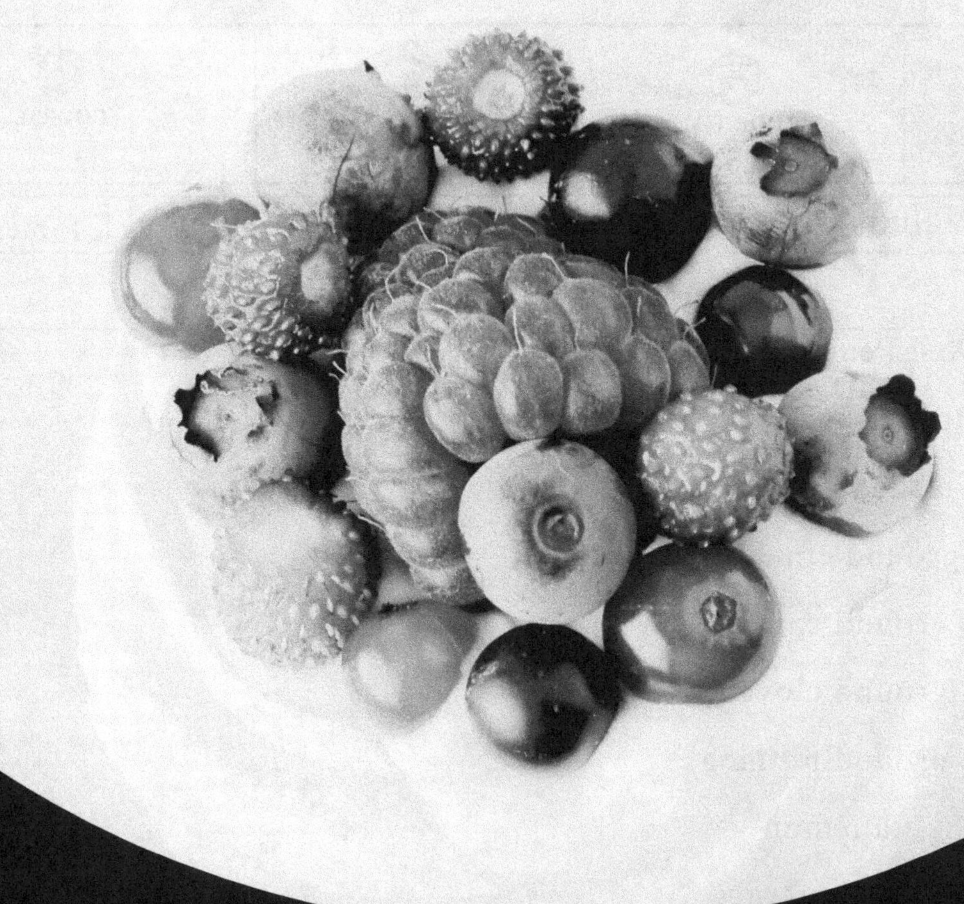

DESSERTS

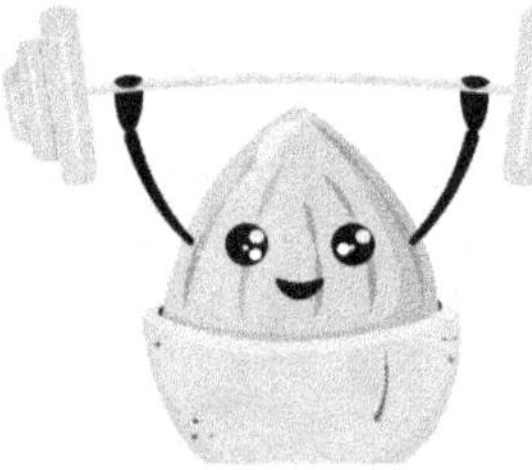

Baked Pears with Almonds, Honey and Ricotta

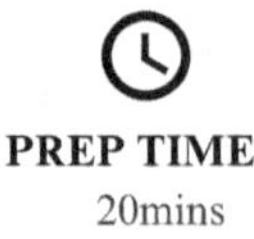

PREP TIME:	COOK TIME:	SERVINGS:	COURSE:
20mins	30mins	12	Dessert

Nutritional Value:	Calories: 103.3kcal	Fat: 2.8g	Carb: 20.2g	Protein: 1.3g

INGREDIENTS:

- **For The Baked Pears**
- 6 medium Bosc pears
- ¼ cup brown sugar
- 1 teaspoon ground cinnamon
- ½ teaspoon ground cardamom
- ¼ teaspoon ground cloves
- ⅛ teaspoon ground nutmeg
- Juice from half a lemon
- 1 teaspoon almond extract

- **For The Candied Nuts (Optional)**
- 2 teaspoons honey
- 1 ¼ teaspoon olive oil
- ½ teaspoon Kosher salt
- ½ cup slivered almonds
- **To Serve**
- Whole milk ricotta cheese
- Honey

DIRECTIONS:

- Preheat the oven to 350 degrees Fahrenheit.

- To prepare the pears, cut them in half and scrape out the rough core and seeds in the center with a spoon.

- Make the sauce: Brown sugar, cinnamon, cardamom, cloves, nutmeg, half a lemon juice, and almond extract should be combined in a 9x13 baking dish. To blend, stir everything together. Make an effort to push it along the bottom of the baking dish so that it forms a thin layer

- Bake the pears: Dip the pears in the brown sugar mixture, cut side down. Cover and bake for 30 minutes, or until a knife inserted into the pear meets no resistance.

- While the pears are baking, combine the honey, olive oil, and salt in a small skillet over medium heat. Swirl the pan a few times before adding the almonds. Stir the almonds around with a rubber spatula to coat them. Cook, stirring periodically, for 6 to 8 minutes, or until fragrant and a deep, golden brown. Keep an eye on them since they can quickly move from toasted to charred. Allow to cool on a plate lined with parchment paper.

- To serve, spoon some ricotta into a shallow bowl and gently distribute it around. Place one or two pear halves cut side up on a plate, spread part of the sauce from the baking dish over the pears, sprinkle with candied almonds, and drizzle with honey.

- In this recipe, I used 6 medium Bosc pears, which fit snugly in the baking dish. It's similar to playing Tetris, but you want to make sure that the cut surface of each pear rests on top of the sugar spice mixture. If necessary, use two baking dishes.

- This recipe is already quite basic, but you can make it even simpler by omitting the nuts.

- I used ricotta cheese because it's not too sweet and helps balance the sugars with fat and protein, but you could also use a dollop of ice cream, whipped cream, or honey-sweetened Greek yogurt.

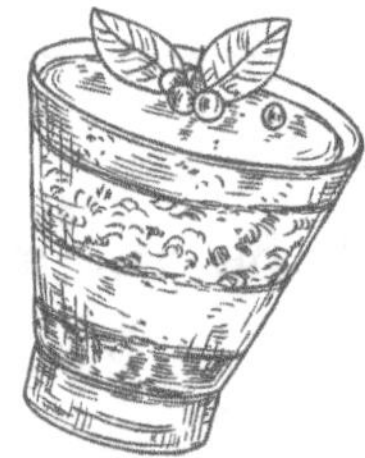

Pumpkin Parfait (Healthy Gluten Free Dessert)

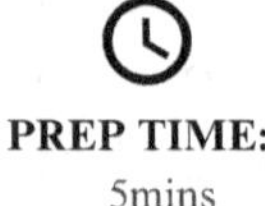 **PREP TIME:** 5mins	 **COOK TIME:** 0min	 **SERVINGS:** 6 servings	 **COURSE:** Dessert

Nutritional Value:	Calories: 143.4kcal	Fat: 4.1g	Carb: 19.5g	Protein: 6.1g

INGREDIENTS:

- 1 15-ounce can pumpkin puree, or scant 2 cups homemade pumpkin puree
- 1 ¼ cup Greek yogurt
- 3-4 tablespoons mascarpone cheese
- 1 tablespoon vanilla extract
- 2 ½ tablespoons brown sugar
- 1 ½-2 teaspoons ground cinnamon
- ¼ teaspoon nutmeg

- **Parfait Toppings**
- 2 tablespoons honey or molasses, more for garnish
- Chocolate chips for garnish
- Chopped hazelnuts or walnuts for garnish

DIRECTIONS:

- In a large mixing bowl, combine the pumpkin puree, Greek yogurt, and all of the remaining ingredients, except the chocolate chips and nuts. Mix everything together with a hand electric mixer or a whisk until it's smooth.

- Taste it and modify the flavor to your desire (for example, add a bit of molasses or brown sugar to sweeten it even more). Alternatively, if you want extra cinnamon or nutmeg, alter the spices.) Mix once more to combine.

- Pour the pumpkin-yogurt mixture into small (3-ounce) goblets or mason jars. Refrigerate for 30 minutes or overnight, covered.

- When ready to serve, drizzle each with molasses and sprinkle with chocolate chips and chopped hazelnuts or walnuts. Enjoy!

NOTES:

- Make-ahead tip: You may make this pumpkin parfait the night before. Refrigerate in an airtight container or individual mason jars (save the chocolate chips and nuts for later). When ready to serve, stir the yogurt mixture and pour it into serving goblets or tiny jars, then proceed to step 3.

- To accommodate a larger group: To feed 12 or more people (small 3-ounce goblets or mason jars), simply double the recipe.

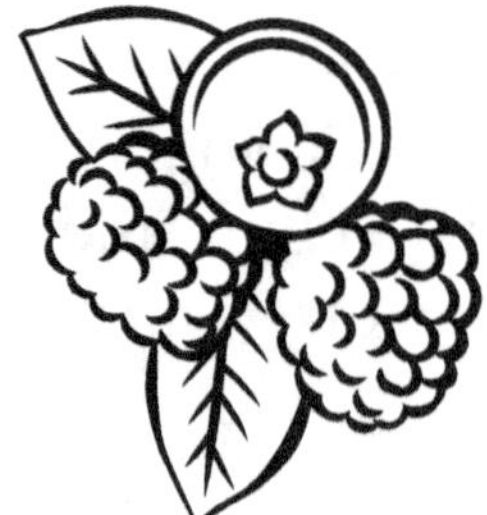

Quick Berry Compote Recipe (5 Ingredients. 2 Ways.)

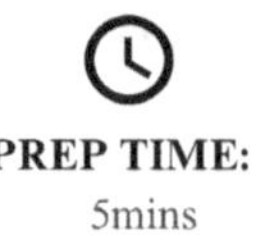 **PREP TIME:** 5mins	 **COOK TIME:** 25mins	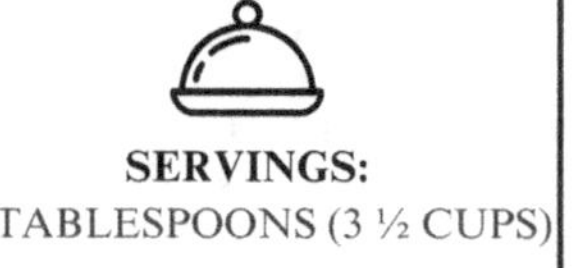 **SERVINGS:** 56 TABLESPOONS (3 ½ CUPS)	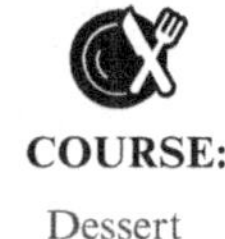 **COURSE:** Dessert

Nutritional Value:	Calories: 10.8kcal	Fat: 0.1g	Carb: 2.7g	Protein: 0.2g

INGREDIENTS:

- 12 ounces fresh strawberries, hulled and chopped
- 12 ounces fresh blueberries
- 12 ounces fresh raspberries
- 3 tablespoons raw cane sugar
- Juice of 1 lime, optional (you can start with juice of ½ lime)

DIRECTIONS:

Stovetop Method

- In a medium skillet or pot, combine the strawberries, blueberries, and raspberries. Combine the sugar and lime juice in a mixing bowl. To mix, toss everything together.

- Bring the mixture to a boil over medium-high heat for about 5 minutes, stirring regularly.

- When the fruit mixture has reached a boil and the sugar has dissolved, reduce the heat to low (the lowest setting on your burner). Allow the berries to boil for 15 to 20 minutes, stirring frequently, until the fruit has softened and the compote has decreased by about a quarter of its volume.

- Take the pan off the heat. If you want a smoother compote, mash the fruit little more with the back of a fork or a potato masher (I prefer bits of fruit in mine). You can also taste to alter the sweetness. I don't normally need to add additional sugar, but if you do, you can sprinkle some more cane sugar or drizzle some honey on top. Make sure to thoroughly combine the ingredients.

- Allow the berry compote to cool for 15–30 minutes before serving. It will thicken further.

Oven Method (Roasted):

- Preheat the oven to 375°F

- Combine the strawberries, blueberries, and raspberries in a large mixing dish. Combine the sugar and lime juice in a mixing bowl. Toss the bananas in the sugar and lime juice to coat.

- Transfer the fruit mixture to a large baking dish or a heavy, rimmed sheet pan, spreading it out evenly in a single layer.

- Cook for 30 to 45 minutes, checking every 10 to 15 minutes, until the berries have collapsed and released some liquids. You may want to remove the baking dish from the oven from time to time to stir the fruit.

- Allow 15 to 20 minutes for the roasted berries to cool before serving.

NOTES:

- Can you make this compote with frozen fruit? Yes, and you don't have to thaw it first. The compote will just take a few minutes longer to cook.

- When the triple berry compote has completely cooled, put it to a mason jar and tightly seal it. Refrigerate for up to 10 days before using.

Melissa Clark's Raspberry Clafouti

 **PREP TIME:** 15mins

 **COOK TIME:** 35mins

 **SERVINGS:** 6 People

 **COURSE:** Dessert

Nutritional Value:	Calories: 135kcal	Fat: 3.9g	Carb: 33.5g	Protein: 5.8g

INGREDIENTS:

- Unsalted butter for baking dish
- 3 cups (350 grams) raspberries
- ½ cup plus 1 tablespoon granulated sugar divided
- 1 teaspoon dried lavender buds (optional)
- ½ cup (120 millilitres) whole milk
- ½ cup (114 grams) crème fraiche, more for serving (optional)
- 4 large eggs
- Pinch salt
- ⅓ cup (43 grams) all-purpose flour
- Confectioners' sugar for serving

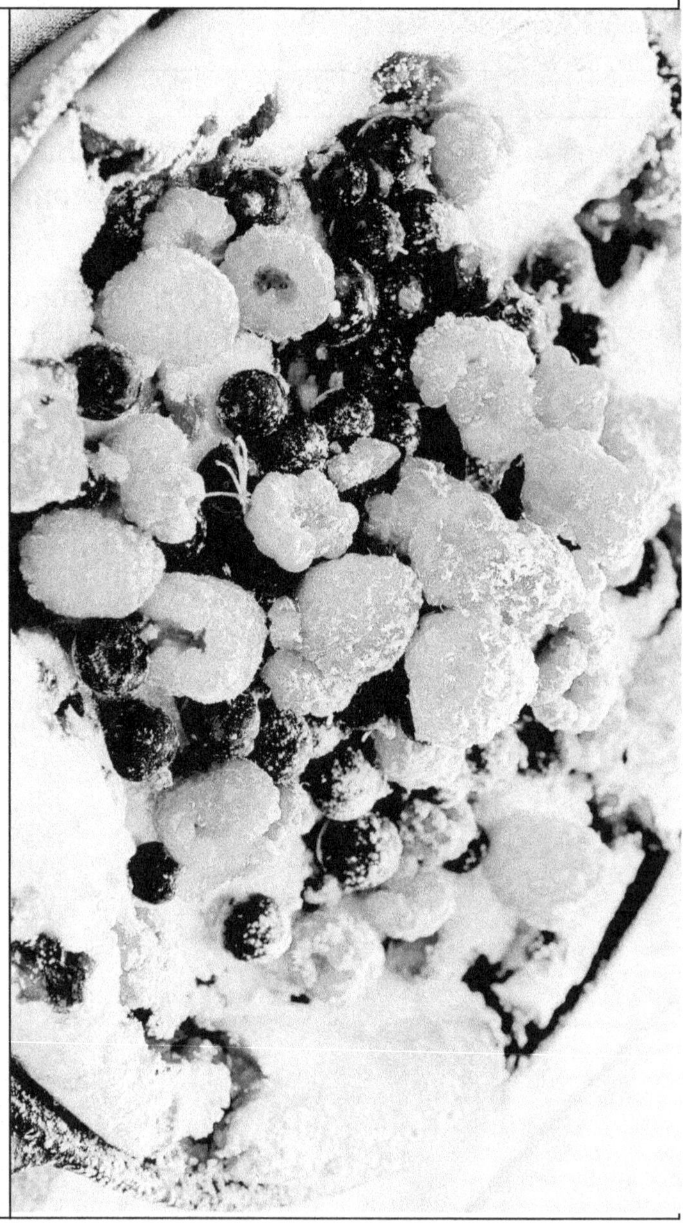

DIRECTIONS:

- Preheat the oven to 375°F. Prepare a 9-inch ceramic baking dish, a 2-quart gratin dish, or a 9- inch cake pan with butter.

- Toss the raspberries with 1 tablespoon sugar in a medium bowl. Allow them to sit while you prepare the rest of the ingredients.

- In a food processor or blender, combine the remaining 12 cup sugar and the lavender; process for 2 minutes, or until the lavender is mostly crushed. Then add the milk, crème fraiche, eggs, and salt and mix well. Simply pulse in the flour to mix.

- Arrange the sugared berries in the prepared baking dish, followed by the egg mixture. Bake for 35 minutes, or until the cake is brown and the middle bounces back when lightly touched.

- Place the baking dish on a wire rack to cool for at least 15 minutes before serving. Then coat it with confectioners' sugar, slice it, and serve it with a dollop of whipped crème fraiche (I served it with Greek yogurt).

NOTES:

- Clafouti is ideally served within an hour of baking, while it is still soft and warm, although it can be served up to 6 hours later (at room temperature).

- You can make this recipe without the lavender buds if you don't have any. It's extremely subtle in this recipe, and I'll probably add a little more next time.

- For baking clafouti, use a ceramic dish. Avoid using metal baking pans, which might cause the edges of the clafouti to burn before they set.

- Leftovers: cover and refrigerate overnight for a delicious breakfast topped with Greek yogurt and additional berries! It is advised that any remaining clafoutis be consumed within 24 hours.

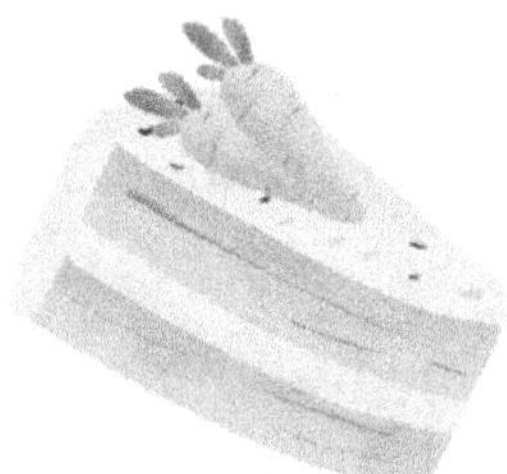

Healthy Carrot Cake Recipe with Honey and Whole Wheat Flour

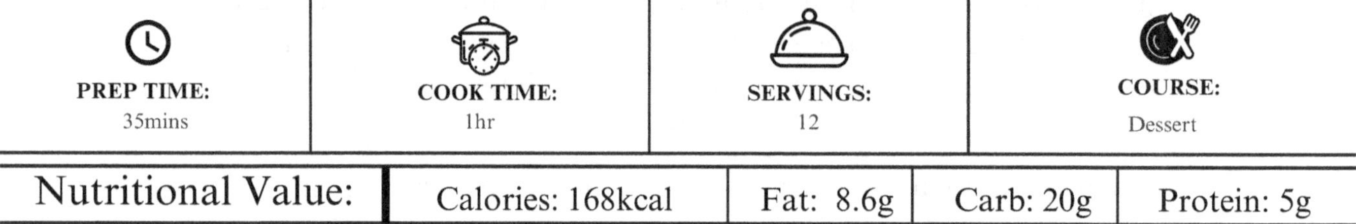

PREP TIME: 35mins	**COOK TIME:** 1hr	**SERVINGS:** 12	**COURSE:** Dessert

Nutritional Value:	Calories: 168kcal	Fat: 8.6g	Carb: 20g	Protein: 5g

INGREDIENTS:

- ½ cup Private Reserve Greek extra virgin olive oil
- ½ cup Greek yogurt (reduced fat)
- ⅓ cup milk (2% reduced fat milk)
- ½ cup quality dark honey
- 3 eggs at room temperature
- 2 ¼ cup whole wheat flour
- 1 ½ tsp baking powder
- ½ tsp salt
- 4 tsp ground cinnamon
- ½ tsp ground cardamom
- ¼ tsp ground ginger
- 2 cups finely grated carrots (you can use food processor to very finely chop instead)
- 6 Medjool dates, pitted and finely chopped (you can use food processor)
- ⅓ cup chopped walnuts
- powdered sugar for light dusting

DIRECTIONS:

- Preheat the oven to 350°F.

- Whisk together the olive oil, geek yogurt, and milk in a large mixing dish. Whisk together the eggs one at a time.

- Separately, whisk together the flour, baking powder, salt, and spices.

- Mix the dry ingredients into the wet ingredients gradually with a wooden spoon.

- Incorporate the carrots. Mix well, then add the dates and walnuts. Mix with the wooden spoon once more until well blended.

- Line a 9-inch square baking pan with parchment paper (or lightly cover with olive oil). Fill the pan halfway with carrot cake batter.

- Bake for 1 hour at 350°F (or until a toothpick put into the center of the cake comes out clean). Allow to cool completely. If desired, top with powdered sugar. Cut the dough into 9 or 12 square pieces. Enjoy!

NOTES:

- Instructions for freezing You can simply freeze this cake if you wish to prepare it for a smaller crowd or for yourself for breakfast.

- Once completely cool, slice the cake into the desired number of pieces; cover and freeze in the baking pan (if freezer safe) or transfer to a freezer safe tray.

- Allow it to freeze until it is solid (approximately 4 hours). Then remove the pieces and wrap them separately in plastic wrap and a final layer of aluminum foil. Refrigerate the items you require overnight.

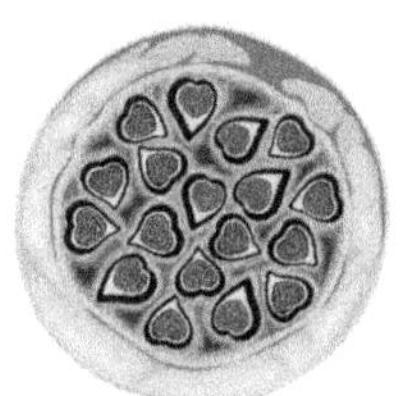

Easy Fig Pastry Recipe

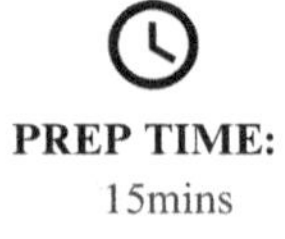			
PREP TIME:	**COOK TIME:**	**SERVINGS:**	**COURSE:**
15mins	20mins	4	Dessert

Nutritional Value:	Calories: 703kcal	Fat: 51.5g	Carb: 47.6g	Protein: 14.1g

INGREDIENTS:

- 1 sheet of good store-bought puff pastry, thawed in fridge for 3 hours or so
- 8 oz fresh black mission figs
- 4-5 oz goat cheese, room temperature
- ¼ cup walnuts, roughly chopped; more for garnish if desired
- 2 tbsp good fig jam
- 1 tbsp butter, melted
- ¼ cup fresh mint leaves, roughly chopped (optional)

DIRECTIONS:

Stovetop Method

- Preheat the oven to 375 degrees Fahrenheit.
- Place four approximately equal rectangular pieces of thawed puff pastry on a baking sheet coated with parchment paper.
- On each piece, spread goat cheese. Then add the jam, figs, and walnuts.
- Brush figs and puff pastry edges with melted butter.
- Turn the pastry edges up slightly.
- Bake for 18-20 minutes at 375°F, or until the pastry is golden and fluffy.
- If preferred, garnish with chopped mint leaves and more walnuts.

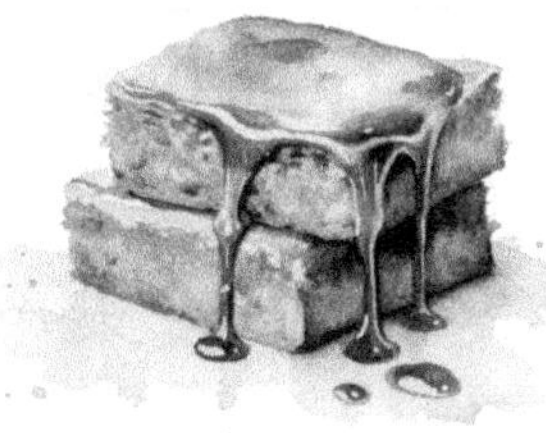

Healthy Black Bean Brownies

 **PREP TIME:** 15mins	 **COOK TIME:** 25mins	 **SERVINGS:** 16	 **COURSE:** Dessert

Nutritional Value:	Calories: 172kcal	Fat: 12g	Carb: 15g	Protein: 3g

INGREDIENTS:

- Black Beans– 1 15 ounce can.

- Unsweetened Cocoa Powder– ¼ cup.

- Baking Powder– 1 teaspoon.

- All Purpose Flour– ¼ cup.

- Banana- 1.

- Chocolate Chips– ½ cup plus additional as desired for topping. Maple Syrup– ¼ cup.

- Canola Oil– ½ cup.

- Vanilla Extract– 1 teaspoon.

- Chopped Nuts– ¾ cup plus additional as desired for topping.

DIRECTIONS:

- Preheat the oven to 350°F and prepare a nonstick baking dish (9 X 13 works nicely). This recipe should work with parchment paper.

- If you haven't previously, rinse the black beans in cool water. Allow the beans to drain after that.

- Whisk or combine the unsweetened cocoa powder, baking powder, and flour in a medium mixing dish.

- Next, in a food processor or excellent blender, combine the beans and chocolate chips until well combined. Then add the banana, syrup, and oil and mix until smooth.

- Process the dry ingredients from the first bowl, together with the vanilla essence, in a food processor until smooth. Then add the chopped nuts.

- Place the prepared baking dish on top of the mixture. Top with extra chocolate chips and almonds if desired. Cook for 20–25 minutes. Allow the brownies to cool completely on a rack before cutting.

NOTES:

- Instead of the customary dairy components used in brownies, this recipe calls for a banana and oil.

- In addition, black beans are included in this brownie recipe, which gives the brownies a thicker, more fudge-like texture.

- I also stated that the black beans should be cooked before being added to this dish.

- A 15-ounce can of black beans is required for this dish. Rinse the black beans in a colander with cool water. Allow the beans to rinse before using in this recipe.

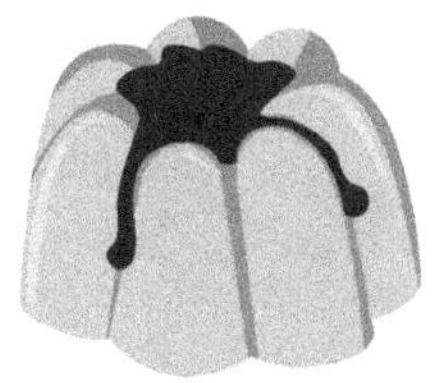

Chocolate Chia Pudding

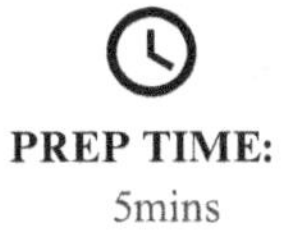 PREP TIME:	 COOK TIME:	 SERVINGS:	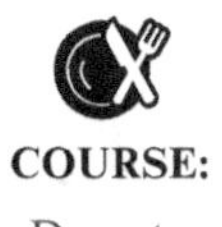 COURSE:
5mins	4hrs	2	Dessert

Nutritional Value:	Calories: 192kcal	Fat: 6g	Carb: 26g	Protein: 5g

INGREDIENTS:

- 2 tablespoons cacao powder
- 2 tablespoons maple syrup
- 1 teaspoon vanilla extract
- 1 cup milk (dairy or dairy-free)
- ¼ cup chia seeds

GARNISH

- raspberries (or other fruit)
- chocolate shavings
- coconut whipped cream
- nuts and seeds

DIRECTIONS:

- Add the cacao powder, maple syrup, vanilla extract, dairy-free milk, and chia seeds to a medium-sized mixing bowl. Whisk until all of the ingredients are incorporated.

- Allow the mixture to stand in the bowl for 15 minutes without stirring to allow the chia seeds to gel. After 15 minutes, mix everything together again. Place the bowl in the refrigerator overnight, or at least 4 hours.

- Take the chocolate chia seed pudding out of the refrigerator and whisk it together with a spoon. Pour into tiny dessert cups. Garnish with your preferred fruit, chocolate shavings, or other garnishes.

NOTES:

- If your chia seeds haven't begun to gel and thicken after 10 minutes, you may have received faulty chia seeds. This is possible if they've been sitting in your pantry for a while. Simply purchase a new bag of chia seeds.

- If you want your berries to seem frosted, follow these steps. Freeze fresh berries that have been cleaned and dried in a single layer on a plate. Once frozen, stir them into the chocolate chia pudding. They'll have that frosted look after about 2 to 3 minutes (when they get to room temperature). But serve them quickly since they won't last long!

Mixed Berry Crisp

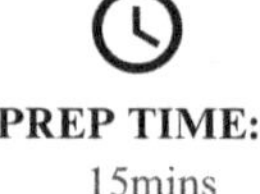 **PREP TIME:** 15mins	 **COOK TIME:** 45mins	 **SERVINGS:** 6 Serving	 **COURSE:** Dessert

Nutritional Value:	Calories: 336kcal	Fat: 11g	Carb: 59g	Protein: 3g

INGREDIENTS:

- 4 tablespoons flour
- 1 teaspoon lemon zest
- ¼ cup sugar
- Topping
- ½ cup brown sugar
- ½ cup oats
- ½ cup coconut
- ¼ cup salted butter softened
- ¼ cup all purpose flour
- ¼ cup chopped pecans (optional)
- ½ teaspoon cinnamon

DIRECTIONS:

- Preheat the oven to 375 degrees Fahrenheit.
- Combine the berries, flour, lemon zest, and sugar in a 2-quart baking dish.
- In a medium mixing bowl, add brown sugar, oats, coconut, butter, flour, chopped pecans (if using), and cinnamon. Sprinkle topping on top of berries.
- 30–35 minutes, or until the berries are heated and bubbling.
- Allow at least 10 minutes to cool before serving. If preferred, top with vanilla ice cream

NOTES:

- If using frozen fruit, increase the cooking time by 15 minutes and add 1 tablespoon more flour. If the topping begins to brown too quickly, cover the dish gently with foil (do not seal the foil, just put it over top).
- Plan ahead of time. Make a double or triple batch of topping and freeze it in individual freezer bags. When a craving comes, simply place the fruit in a baking dish and top with the frozen topping.

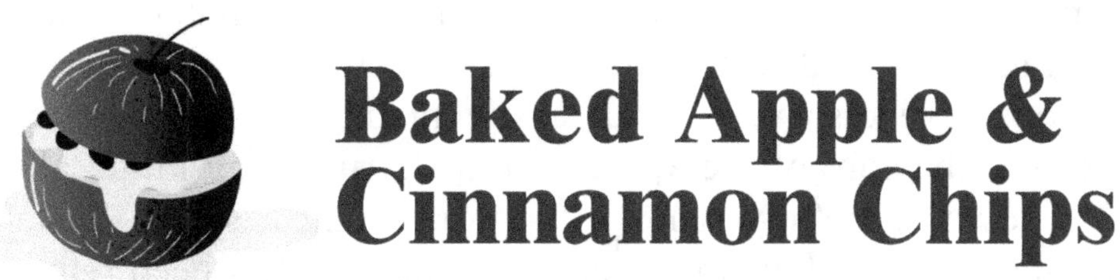

Baked Apple & Cinnamon Chips

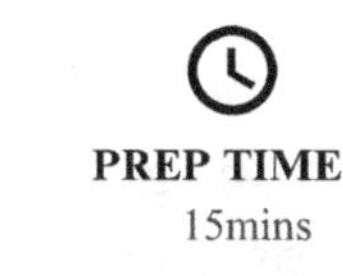			
PREP TIME: 15mins	**COOK TIME:** 45mins	**SERVINGS:** 4	**COURSE:** Dessert

Nutritional Value:	Calories: 52kcal	Fat: 0.2g	Carb: 14g	Protein: 0.3g

INGREDIENTS:

- 3 Tablespoons (43g) unsalted butter, softened to room temperature (extra soft, so it's easy to mash)
- 1/4 cup (50g) packed light or dark brown sugar
- 1/2 teaspoon ground cinnamon
- 1/8 teaspoon ground nutmeg
- 1/4 cup (21g) old-fashioned whole rolled oats
- 4 large apples (see note), rinsed and patted dry
- optional: 2 Tablespoons raisins, dried cranberries, or chopped nuts
- For Baking
- 3/4 cup (180ml) warm water

DIRECTIONS:

- Preheat the oven to 375 degrees Fahrenheit (191 degrees Celsius).
- Beat/mash the butter, sugar, cinnamon, and nutmeg together with a fork or spoon, or a handheld or stand mixer fitted with a paddle attachment. Stir in the oats and, if using, the raisins/dried cranberries/nuts. Place aside.

- Apple corer: This can be difficult, but I recommend using a sharp paring knife and a spoon. (Alternatively, an apple corer.) Cookie scoops, I've discovered, can easily break or crack the apples. Cut around the core of the apple with a sharp paring knife, about 1/2 or 3/4 down. Carefully remove the core using a spoon. It takes some perseverance and arm muscle. Once the core has been removed, use a spoon to extract any remaining seeds.

- Fill an 8-inch or 9-inch baking pan, cake pan, or pie dish halfway with cored apples. Fill each apple all the way to the top with filling. Pour heated water around the apples in the pan. Water keeps the apples from drying out and scorching.

- Bake for 40-45 minutes, or until apples are tender. Longer baking time results in softer, mushier baked apples. The time required is determined by how firm your apples were and how soft you want them to be.

- Remove the apples from the oven and, if desired, baste the outside with pan juices. This gives moisture to the skin, but it is entirely optional.

- Warm with salted caramel, whipped cream, or ice cream on top. Refrigerate leftovers for up to 2 days after cooking.

NOTES:

- Instructions for Making Ahead: I don't recommend making the baked apples ahead of time to serve later. They quickly discolor and become mushy. Instead, make the filling ahead of time, cover it, and chill it for up to 3 days before spooning it into the apples and baking them. I don't advocate freezing these baked apples since they thaw out too mushy.

- Best Apples to Use: Choose apples that are precisely round and solid. Granny Smith, Fuji, Pink Lady, or Honeycrisp apples are my favorites. To avoid tipping over in the oven, make sure they stand up straight on their bottoms.

- Brown sugar provides moisture as well as the best flavor. If necessary, add regular granulated sugar or even coconut sugar. I do not advocate any liquid sweeteners or sugar substitutes.

- Oatmeal: Oatmeal adds a lovely texture. You can substitute quick oats for the same quantity. I don't recommend cutting out the oats, but if you must, finely chopped nuts can be substituted. I do not recommend substituting oat flour or any other flour.

CONCLUSION

As we near the end of "Mediterranean Diet for Beginners 2024," let's recap the fundamental themes that make this culinary trip both enriching and transformative for novices.

Recap of Key Points:

- The key to success is to embrace the simplicity of fresh, whole foods. Allow the brilliant colors and flavors of fruits and vegetables, whole grains, and lean proteins to guide your culinary adventure.

- Versatility for All Tastes: Whether you enjoy savory seafood, robust grains, or brilliant salads, the Mediterranean diet has something for everyone. Experiment to find out what makes you happy.

- Healthy Fats, Wholesome Proteins: Highlight the benefits of healthy fats such as olive oil, nuts, and seeds, as well as wholesome proteins such as fish, lentils, and lean meats. These are the foundations of a healthy Mediterranean diet.

- Moderation and Balance: Limit portion amounts and savor each bite attentively. The Mediterranean way of life emphasizes balance over deprivation.

- Culinary Experimentation: Make the kitchen your playground. Experiment with different herbs, spices, and ingredients. The Mediterranean diet encourages you to appreciate the cooking process as much as the joys of the table.

Tips for Beginners:

- Begin slowly: Include a couple Mediterranean-inspired meals in your weekly routine. As you become more familiar with the ingredients and flavors, gradually broaden your repertory.

- Plan and prep: To make the cooking process easier, plan your meals ahead of time and perform some meal prep. Having important items on hand can transform a stressful day into a stressfree culinary experience.

- Shared Meals: Enjoy the social side of dining. Share your Mediterranean-inspired dishes with family and friends to build community around the table.

Encouragement for Long-Term Success:

- Choosing the Mediterranean diet is a commitment to long-term well-being, not just short-term adjustments. Here are some words of encouragement for your continued success:

- Celebrate Progress: Each step along the way is a win. Celebrate the beneficial changes in your food habits and entire lifestyle.

- Pay Attention to Your Body: Pay attention to how your body reacts to various foods. The Mediterranean diet is all about feeding your body in a way that feels good to you.

- Make it Your Own: Tailor the Mediterranean diet to your tastes and lifestyle. Find methods to make your journey uniquely yours, whether you're a vegetarian, vegan, or have special nutritional demands.

- Continue to be Curious: Keep trying different recipes, ingredients, and cooking techniques. The Mediterranean diet is a culinary experience that evolves and surprises you on a regular basis.

As you finish this book, keep in mind that the Mediterranean diet is not a fixed set of rules, but rather a way of life that changes with you. May your path be blessed with savory discoveries, bright health, and the lasting delight that comes from learning to live well.

I Have a Request

We hope you liked Janie Stafford's "Mediterranean Diet for Beginners 2024" gastronomic excursion. Your experience and feedback are extremely valuable to us!

If this book has improved the taste of your kitchen and the wellbeing of your life, we ask you to share your ideas and insights by writing a review. Your reviews not only offer us with vital input, but they also help fellow readers who are thinking about embarking on this Mediterranean gastronomic trip.

Here are a few prompts to consider:

- *What recipes did you find most delightful and why?*
- *How has the simplicity of the book helped you, especially if you're a beginner in the Mediterranean*
- *diet?*
- *Have you experienced any positive changes in your eating habits or well-being since incorporating*
- *these recipes into your routine?*

Your honest reviews help us continue crafting meaningful content and inspire others to embrace
a healthier, more flavorful lifestyle.

Thank you for being a part of our culinary community, and we look forward to hearing about your Mediterranean diet journey!

Happy Cooking,
The Team at Janie Stafford's Kitchen

9 798876 413284